Yoga for One

of related interest

Restorative Yoga
Power, Presence and Practice for Teachers and Trainees
Anna Ashby
Foreword by Richard Rosen
ISBN 978 1 78775 739 4
eISBN 978 1 78775 740 0
Audio ISBN 978 1 52937 102 4

Teaching Body-Positive Yoga
A Guide to Language, Inclusivity and Props
Donna Noble
Foreword by Jivana Heyman
ISBN 978 1 78775 335 8
eISBN 978 1 78775 336 5

The Online Yoga Teacher's Guide
Get Confident and Thrive Online
Jade Beckett
ISBN 978 1 83997 180 8
eISBN 978 1 83997 181 5

Chair Yoga
Seated Exercises for Health and Wellbeing
Edeltraud Rohnfeld
ISBN 978 1 84819 078 8
eISBN 978 0 85701 056 8

YOGA for ONE

How to Co-Create an Inclusive and Evidence-Informed Practice On and Off the Mat

Suzie Carmack, PhD, MFA, MEd,
ERYT 500, NBC-HWC, C-IAYT, PCC

Forewords by
Dr. Avinash Patwardhan and Alyssa Wostrel

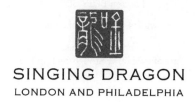

SINGING DRAGON
LONDON AND PHILADELPHIA

First published in Great Britain in 2024 by Singing Dragon, an imprint of Jessica Kingsley Publishers
Part of John Murray Press

2

Figure 2: Used with permission of Elsevier Science & Technology Journals, from Social
Science & Medicine, From policy to patient: Using a socio-ecological framework to
explore the factors influencing safe practice in UK primary care, Litchfield, Ian; Perryman,
Katherine; Avery, Anthony; Campbell, Stephen; Gill, Paramjit; Greenfield, Sheila, vol. 277
p. 113906 © 2021; permission conveyed through Copyright Clearance Center, Inc.
Figure 6: Copyright © 2012 by (SAGE Publications) Reprinted by Permission of SAGE Publications
Figure 7: Used with permission of REAL Wellness LLC, from AWR 641 – Jack Travis, M.D. and the
Illness/Wellness Continuum – 3-12-2013, Key Concept #1: The Illness-Wellness Continuum, John
Travis Sara Ryan, © 2013; permission conveyed through Copyright Clearance Center, Inc.

Front cover image source: Kris Meade, Meade Agency. The cover image is for
illustrative purposes only, and any person featuring is a model.

Photography by Kris Meade and David Stinzi, Meade Agency, and Attimi Guillermo, Attimi Photography.

A CIP catalogue record for this title is available from the British Library and the Library of Congress

ISBN 978 1 80501 025 8
eISBN 978 1 80501 026 5

Printed and bound by CPI Group (UK) Ltd, Croydon, CR0 4YY

Jessica Kingsley Publishers' policy is to use papers that are natural, renewable and recyclable
products and made from wood grown in sustainable forests. The logging and manufacturing
processes are expected to conform to the environmental regulations of the country of origin.

Singing Dragon
Carmelite House
50 Victoria Embankment
London EC4Y 0DZ

www.singingdragon.com

John Murray Press
Part of Hodder & Stoughton Limited
An Hachette UK Company

Contents

Foreword by Dr. Avinash Patwardhan 7

Foreword by Alyssa Wostrel 9

Acknowledgments 11

Prologue 13

1. Why Yoga for One? 15

2. Co-Creating Evidence-Informed Person-Centered Care 31

3. Building Your Program Foundation with a Business Model 55

4. Social Marketing: An Inclusive Approach to Your Marketing Mix 77

5. Meeting the Client Where They Are: Assessment Tools 101

6. Co-Creating an Evidence-Informed Program Plan 203

7. Aligning Daily Practices to the Program Needs and Goals:
   Inclusive Strategies 221

About the Author 253

Endnotes 255

Figures

Figure 1: Yoga for One evidence-informed 3 Es model 32

Figure 2: Socio-ecological framework showing the influences on patient safety in primary care 37

Figure 3: Yoga for One business model 57

Figure 4: Yoga for One 9 Ps of the marketing mix 78

Figure 5: Yoga for One value ladder 89

Figure 6: Sense-making theory by Dervin 157

Figure 7: The wellness continuum 168

Figure 8: Yoga for One program logic model 210

Tables

Table 1: Person-centered care outcomes 46

Table 2: Vata, pitta, and kapha imbalances in the koshas 119

Table 3: Overview of the traffic light method 169

Foreword by Dr. Avinash Patwardhan

क्षुरस्य धारा निशिता दुरत्यया ("attaining yoga salvation") is like walking on the sharp edge of a razor, so says one of the oldest references to yoga in Sanskrit scriptures of ancient India. To write a book on yoga, and then particularly addressing yogis themselves regarding how to professionally conduct and manage yoga teaching to help their clients climb the same difficult mountain of health and well-being, alongside and within a falling Niagara of books and articles on yoga all around, is a tall order to say the least. Therefore, when Dr. Carmack, my friend Suzie, approached me with a request to write a foreword for her book, I was skeptical and told her that I would read through the book, and if I felt that it was measuring up, then and only then I would take to pen. Suzie not only walked the walk but also did it like that ballerina that she was once in her previous life. Lately it has become fashionable to paint yoga in bright, glorious colors, and portray it larger than life size. Against that background, Dr. Carmack pointing out politely, but firmly, that "yoga is not easy," or that on average societal "yoga literacy" is low, or that yoga professionals' own "ego and mistaken assumptions (regarding yoga) can be a barrier" for the teacher as well as the client to attain yoga benefits, or that if not managed carefully and well, "yoga can do more harm than help," are not only refreshing thoughts but are very timely, apt, and of indubitable value in current times, when stress and mental health issues and chronic diseases are siphoning away the benefits that the advances in modern sciences and technologies offer, and where the socio-political environment is becoming increasingly unnerving, not only to the already weak and suffering, but even to those who are relatively more fortunate.

Another thing that I find laudable in the book is the discussion about managing the "business of yoga" or the "monetizing of services" without carrying the burden of guilt of feeling oneself, in Dr. Carmack's words, "sold out." Few books, to my knowledge, attempt to tackle this onerous but necessary topic because, on the face of it, the practice of yoga, of care compassion and spirituality, and the business of yoga, does seem like an oxymoron.

The list of pearls of wisdom in this book is long. The "SOAP" framework for evaluation for making a customized program for the client, the foundational principle of co-creation of a program with the client's participation, the essential skill of the art of communication above anything, attention to formalities like waivers, consent, or Health Insurance Portability and Accountability Act (HIPAA) privacy issues, even though currently not mandated by law, and last, but not the least, a wise safety-inclined traffic light method for teaching "postures" are just a few examples.

In the end, someone might wonder as to how and why Dr. Carmack accomplished the daunting task of writing this book, and why one should trust and follow her crumbs. Here is my brief answer to that. I have known Suzie for four+ years. Apart from being a highly educated academic, and being blessed, she has also seen excruciating pain and agony in life, and, as Robert Frost would say, "that has made all the difference."

Dr. Avinash Patwardhan, MD, MS, ERYT500, R CHES, R Fellow AIS
Retired obstetrician-gynecologist; Advisory Committee Member, Integrated Health
Services, World Health Organization (WHO) (2020–present); Committee Member,
WHO Collaborating Centre for Traditional, Complementary and Integrative
Medicine (Yoga), Ministry of Ayush, Government of India (2023–present);
author of seven seminal articles on yoga and public health (2016–17)

Foreword by Alyssa Wostrel

As Executive Director with the International Association of Yoga Therapists (IAYT), I've had the privilege of connecting with numerous yoga professionals deeply dedicated to advancing positive change in the world. Dr. Suzie Carmack is one of those individuals. Dr. Carmack is a visionary with a creative spirit who I met early in her tenure as Department Chair of Yoga Therapy and Ayurveda (YTA) for the Maryland University of Integrative Health (MUIH). I immediately resonated with her energy, humility, and humor, while also appreciating her talent for elucidating strategic opportunities by recognizing what might be missing from the bigger, systems-level picture.

Dr. Carmack's profound expertise, complemented by her extensive wisdom and knowledge with a PhD in health communication, and as a board-certified health and wellness coach (NBC-HWC), and certified yoga therapist (C-IAYT) is showcased in this, her latest book for yoga professionals, *Yoga for One*.

Offering a comprehensive guide, *Yoga for One* equips yoga professionals with a road map to integrate diverse frameworks and business models, spanning from individual practices to societal and community perspectives. This invaluable resource empowers both novice and experienced yoga professionals, fostering their success by anchoring their businesses, ultimately contributing to the thriving well-being of their clients. This inclusive approach establishes a forward pathway that connects all aspects, presenting a holistic solution for the benefit of the entire yoga community.

The brilliance of *Yoga for One* lies in its comprehensive approach. Dr. Carmack defines the intended audience—be it yoga coaches, mentors, teachers, or therapists—and assumes a certain level of yoga knowledge and training in the reader. From this foundation, she imparts a wealth of wisdom and guidance, offering valuable insights that can assist many yoga professionals in establishing and enhancing their businesses and practices. Emphasizing the importance of the yoga professional to embrace an expansive marketing approach (the 9 Ps) in order to create sustainability, Dr. Carmack encourages the reader to engage in their unique marketing message on a deeper level—that of realizing that the process of healing begins with the connection by the future client to the marketing message itself.

At the heart of *Yoga for One* is the idea that yoga professionals collaborate with their clients to craft a personalized experience rooted in authentic and meaningful human connection. This foundational concept is strengthened by an inclusive framework that advocates for an evidence-informed perspective, prioritizing the client's lived experience. Dr. Carmack goes further to integrate a public health orientation into the "Yoga for One" concept, encompassing population health, prevention, education, and awareness through the socio-ecological model. The ripple effect of this intervention extends the positive impact across various levels.

Whether you're a healthcare professional, yoga teacher, coach, therapist, or allied professional—regardless of whether you're in the early or later stages of your career—this book provides valuable insights for you. Whether it's the uplifting inspiration it conveys about the profound wisdom of yoga, or the practical strategies for establishing your business from the ground up, *Yoga for One* is a valuable read. Invest time in absorbing and integrating its methodology into both your personal and professional pursuits, and experience the positive ripple effect for the greater good of the collective.

Alyssa Wostrel, MBA
Executive Director, International Association of Yoga Therapists (2020–present);
Former Executive Director, Integrative Health Policy Consortium (2012–16)

Acknowledgments

Thank you to my family and friends (both living and in heaven) for always being there for me and for loving me in my Truth.

Thank you to my colleagues, team, and students at Maryland University of Integrative Health for your commitment to advancing the fields of yoga therapy and Ayurveda.

Thank you to my team and community at YogaMedCo, especially Alexis Hartwick, for bringing your genius and compassion to your communities.

Thank you to my colleagues at George Mason University Center for the Advancement of Well-Being and College of Public Health, for our ongoing collaborations to advance well-being.

Thank you to my clients over the past 23 years for the honor of being able to support you in your yoga journey within.

Thank you to Attimi Photography and Meade Agency for their photography support, and thanks to the models you see on the cover and in this book: Sharon Arndt, Lelani Busby, Christina Collins-Smith, Jacquayle Dailey, Stefan Goldberg, Warren Graff, Debbie Griffiths, Marcia Faith Jones, Kathleeen Malon, Kathryn Martin, Teri Miles, Teri Noffsinger, Marie Polanco, Phyllis Strand, Joshua Sutherfield, Serena Sutherfield, Megan Tally, Jessica Turner, Cody Whittenburg, Melissa Wilson, and Amy Wiseman.

Special thanks to my family here in my earth school (Dad, Jane, Chris, Brandon, Sophia, Devon, Brian, Levi, and CJ) and my angels Dixie, Cyndi, Pattie, and Eddie.

And most of all...

Thank you to Bob,

For being the One.

Prologue

Many years ago I learned that the joy yoga offers me is not to be found on the mat next to me. I find it somewhere within me, in the midst of a moment of awe, when I am able to clear my Self from my human blocks and witness my Self as part of a larger humanity. Here I feel a union with all that is, all that has been known, and all there is to know. We are one.

But yoga isn't always rainbows and butterflies, in the day-to-days of life. Yoga is hard—and I am not talking about the fancier asanas or the more complicated chants. Yoga is hard because it asks us to ask more of ourselves—not in an ego-driven way, but in a holistic way.

My personal love for yoga has led me to a professional commitment to sharing it, for well over half of my time so far, here, in earth school. I started practicing and studying yoga in my late 20s, as a young mother. I am now a grandmother, well into my 50s. Yoga has been with me through times that were great, times that sucked, and all of the times in between. Somehow I find myself today, after many plot twists in my life, professionally serving as a department chair of Yoga Therapy and Ayurveda for the Maryland University of Integrative Health; as a senior scholar for the Center for the Advancement of Well-Being at George Mason University; and as CEO and founder of a global training company, YogaMedCo. I am also Blessed to love my life as a married mom of three children and two bonus children, and to be a grandmother of two. Yoga is the constant that enables me to show up in so many ways in the world, because it grounds me in the opportunity to show up for myself first.

Before the plot twists of the day can get to me, my yoga helps me to get in touch with me.

This book grew out of my desire to share the love I have for the practice of yoga, and for sharing it in one-on-one sessions. I believe that the world needs yoga more than ever, and that one-on-one work offers a unique value that the public doesn't yet know about or can't afford. I hope to change that through this book.

Thank you for your willingness to join me on this learning journey. Before we begin, I invite you to join me in setting a few intentions for our travels:

Let's care for ourselves so we have the stamina to show up and Serve the greater good.

Let's lean into the mystery that Source has put us here for reasons beyond our understanding.

Let's partner with our clients so we can support them in the process of their self-liberation.

Let's stay grounded in knowing that the truth is already within the client—we are here for them.

And let's not forget to listen to the wisdom of our inner genius—a Source within us all.

Namaste ~

CHAPTER 1

Why Yoga for One?

Let's start with a question:

What does *yoga* mean to you?

Although I can't hear your answer, because this is a book after all, I will start by saying that it has been my experience that there are many interpretations for the word "yoga." Some practitioners and professionals see yoga as the path that we travel within the broader journey of our lives to discover our dharma, while others think of yoga as the actual journey to self-liberation. Yoga is a practice, like music or golf, and yet yoga is also a state of eudaimonic well-being,[1] or being-ness, that we can access with or without practices. Yoga is a philosophy for living, a set of ethical guidelines, a practice of postures, a method for energy attunement, a set of mindfulness activities, and a sacred geometry (yantra). Yoga is a science of the mind, "a philosophy of healing through the conscious focusing of the mind."[2] Yoga is the path to kaivalya—the consciousness that an individual realizes in the seeing of the Self as separate from, and yet in unity with, all there is. These are just a few of the meanings that come up for me, in answer to the question, "What does yoga mean to you?"

Academically speaking, the field, discipline, and practice of yoga defy convention by being at once an art, a science, and a humanities modality, all rolled into one. Yoga invites multiple ways of knowing and crosses many bodies of knowledge. Yoga is an experiential science (in both the natural sciences and the social sciences), because we can empirically study its mechanisms and its impact on humans (individually and collectively). Yoga is a visual and performing art form, as it invites the interpretive and artistic practices of self-examination, self-realization, and creative expression. Yoga is a forum for the humanities—through yoga we can learn much about the history of civilization and the cultural beliefs and civic practices of humans, and critically examine patterns of the human condition.

And yet, even while yoga can be seen as multi-disciplinary, yoga also reaches above and beyond all of these academic areas of inquiry as a trans-disciplinary field. Yoga is beyond our comprehension and collective consciousness, both literally and figuratively; its study asks us to transcend our current understanding of ourselves, and to see ourselves and our human race from a salutogenic lens—one that is less concerned with fragmentation, categorization, and problems, and instead more focused on the coherence, meaning, and manageability of life.

In addition to these conceptual understandings of yoga, I also have my own lived experience of "what yoga means to me." In my life, yoga offers an always-available pause button in the never-ending demands of the day. Here I can notice my feelings about, and my reactions to, whatever the day is asking of me. Through whatever practice or practices I choose on a given day, I am able to pause long enough to check in within myself and with my Self. Yoga grounds me in the knowing that I am not alone in my humanity while it also elevates me above the plot twists of my own very messy human lived experience. Yoga inspires me to care for my human performance system through the practice of lifestyle medicine—in the ways I eat, sleep, exercise, and connect with others—and to remember that I have the pen of my life story. And when I get too caught up in my own human stuff, yoga reminds me that my inner world is connected to a much bigger one that is filled with other humans that I get to experience earth school with. Yoga is a dance I can do whether or not anyone else is watching—a dance within myself, with my Self.

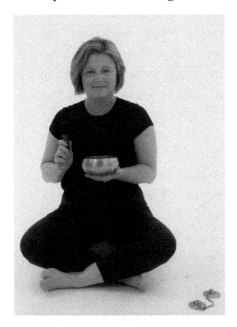

Recognizing that these are just some of the meanings that come up when I personally hear the term "yoga," while also recognizing that you may have more of your own to add here, I would like to acknowledge that there is a beauty and a power in recognizing that each person gets to decide what yoga means to them within these themes. That said, I do find that there is a growing misunderstanding in contemporary popular culture about yoga. Many people believe that yoga is a regimen of physical postures and that it is a practice meant for the privileged, the thin, and the young. Unfortunately, this belief is based on misunderstandings propagated by media depictions of yoga practitioners and the colonization of yoga over time, which has fooled many into the false belief that yoga is a fad for the few when it is, in fact, a tradition for all.

Through this book, I hope to do my best to address this misunderstanding in a novel way. By encouraging yoga professionals to dedicate a portion of their time to co-creating inclusive and evidence-informed programs with their students, clients, or patients, we can shift public perception one human at a time. I would like nothing more than to see the public perception of yoga shift from its current limiting beliefs towards a more limitless understanding.

A VERY BRIEF LOOK BACK ON MY YOGA TEACHING JOURNEY

When I first started teaching yoga (in the late 1990s), I approached it in the same way that I myself had learned it. I told my students and clients what to do and how to do it, and did not invite discussion. Yoga teaching was more about my performance of postures than it was about my actually listening to, and truly seeing, the humans standing right in front of me. We were all caught up in external appearances and ideals of what I thought the practice was supposed to be. Yoga became a regimen and a technique for my students to master and perform—much like the ballet classes I studied when I was very young. My ego fooled me into the false assumption that yoga was about performing (and perfecting) the practice.

I didn't know then what it would take many years of showing up on my mat to discover: yoga isn't just a series of postures, practices, or philosophies. Yoga is a process of self-liberation that unites (connects) us with the rest of the human race and the natural order of the universe. Yoga practices take us on a journey of inner exploration, in which we excavate our Self and our Source to access yoga. When the driving force beneath our yoga practices points inward, we are heading in the right direction of where our inner Truth can be found. But when the driving force beneath our yoga practice aims us outward, into the competitive and judgmental landscape of worldly expectations, we will never find the yoga that was within us all along.

This is why I wish I could go back in time and let the humans who were my early students know that I am sorry I took them to a yoga place that wasn't so yogic after all. But that is not possible. So the best that I can do is to make this right—with the students of my early days of performance teaching and with myself—by sharing some of what I know now to be true. Simply put, I want the yoga teachers, yoga trainers, yoga therapists, and allied health professionals who read this book to learn from my previously unknown and mistaken assumptions. Through this book, I want to invite my yoga colleagues to join me in bringing more yoga into the profession of delivering it.

THE VISION FOR YOGA FOR ONE

In this ideal state (vision), yoga professionals spend less time talking at the humans standing in front of them and more time asking them what they notice within themselves. They spend more time acknowledging how the student, client, or patient is showing up for their own hero's journey, and less time pointing out what is wrong with their mind, body, heart, or spirit. They spend more time supporting the human in the healing of their life story, and less time trying to manage their medical chart. They spend more time listening to their student, client, or patient as they access their inner knowing and intuition, and less time pointing out what their student, client, or patient doesn't know. They spend more time helping their clients to access the gifts and joy of self-liberation, and less time confining themselves or their clients to the standards of a given yoga style.

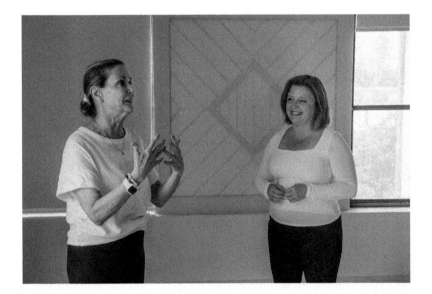

If this vision is one that you are open to, then consider this as your invitation to join me on this journey. This book will teach you the methodology and techniques I have developed for co-creating a Yoga for One program for clients on and off the mat.[3] You are invited to integrate the methodology and the techniques into your own approach in a way that works well for you and your clients. If, along the way, you get lost in the methodology or discover a technique that doesn't work for you and/or your clients, please recalibrate to the vision we are aiming for together as our north star. When in doubt, remember that the client has the answers within, and that this journey is ultimately about them. We are here to co-create a practice with them and for them, in a way that brings them back to their inner truth. It really is all about them—not us.

WHAT ARE THE INTENTIONS OF A YOGA FOR ONE PROGRAM?

We begin this journey like you might begin a yoga class, by setting out the intentions of the Yoga for One program. I invite you to join me in these following intentions, and to decide which one(s) resonates for you. I hope that at least one of these resonates for you so you can find your own "why" for sharing a yoga program with clients in one-on-one programs designed to support them on or off the mat.

Intention 1: Yoga for One promotes inclusivity

My first intention for the Yoga for One program is to promote diversity, equity, inclusion, access, and belonging (otherwise referred to as DEIAB). As yoga spreads across diverse cultures and communities, we can explore how these principles intersect with the delivery of one-on-one yoga:

- *Diversity:* Diversity acknowledges the presence of a wide range of backgrounds, identities, abilities, and perspectives within the yoga community. Yoga studios and classes should reflect this diversity, welcoming individuals of all races, ethnicities, genders, ages, abilities, and socio-economic backgrounds. Through one-on-one yoga programs, we can help individual clients to become more comfortable with yoga so that they can learn that yoga is not a one-size-fits-all practice. By meeting them in their diverse needs, we can support them in finding adaptations that work well for them.

- *Equity:* Equity in yoga ensures that everyone has access to the benefits and opportunities that yoga offers, regardless of their background or circumstances. This includes addressing systemic barriers that may limit access to yoga, such as economic disparities or physical limitations. Through third party funding support for yoga programs, we can bring one-on-one yoga to individuals who might not otherwise be able to afford it.

- *Inclusion:* Inclusion is about creating a sense of belonging and respect for all practitioners, regardless of their differences. In an inclusive yoga space, individuals feel valued, heard, and seen, fostering a sense of unity and shared purpose. A one-on-one yoga program can support both the client and the yoga professional in learning the unique preferences and challenges that individuals face. These insights can then help the yoga professional to know how to co-create a more inclusive training environment with the client, while also building the yoga professional's capacity for leading more inclusive classes.

- *Access:* Yoga can be accessible to everyone, regardless of physical abilities, financial resources, or geographic location. This includes making accommodations for individuals with disabilities and offering affordable or free classes to underserved communities. Through one-on-one yoga programs, the yoga professional can support each individual's accommodation needs to the degree appropriate for the yoga professional's scope of practice.

- *Belonging*: Belonging goes beyond inclusion—it means feeling deeply connected and part of a community. Yoga studios and practitioners can actively foster a sense of belonging where individuals feel at home, safe, and supported. Through one-on-one yoga program support, yoga professionals can support their clients in feeling safe, supported, and secure in their practice.

Yoga has the potential to bring diverse individuals and communities together, fostering a sense of belonging and connection to something greater than the individual or community. In the interaction of a one-on-one setting for the delivery of yoga, we are able to further advance DEIAB principles. We can support the client in sharing their beliefs about themselves on the mat and the challenges they face in their lives off the mat. We can modify the practice in unique ways that are tailored to the specific concerns of the clients' bodies, minds, hearts, spirits, and lives. We have the time and space to focus the delivery of healing presence in a conscious way, and to invite the human to share how this presence feels for them. We can encourage them to share what does and doesn't work for them in their study of yoga philosophy, practices, and postures, and adapt these based on this feedback. We can witness them in their inner exploration and excavation, and encourage them to seek additional supports (referrals and/or resources) if they are beyond the scope of our professional capacity.

Yoga is often celebrated for its ability to bring people of diverse backgrounds, abilities, and identities together in a shared practice. However, achieving true inclusivity in yoga spaces requires conscious effort and a commitment to breaking down barriers. Inclusivity in yoga is essential because it aligns with the core principles of the practice, which emphasize unity, compassion, and connection.

Here are some key reasons why inclusivity is vital:

- *Unity*: Yoga philosophy teaches that we are all interconnected and that our individual experiences are part of a larger whole. Inclusivity fosters a sense of unity, allowing practitioners to experience this interconnectedness firsthand.

- *Respect for diversity*: Yoga recognizes the beauty and value of diversity. Inclusivity honors the uniqueness of each individual, and celebrates the richness of different backgrounds, experiences, and identities.

- *Accessibility*: Inclusivity ensures that yoga is accessible to everyone, regardless of their physical abilities, body size, age, gender, race, or socio-economic status. Yoga should be a practice that meets people where they are.

- *Empowerment:* Inclusivity empowers individuals to embrace their authentic selves and feel a sense of belonging. It encourages practitioners to be confident and self-accepting.

Inclusivity in yoga is not just an aspiration; it is a reflection of the true spirit of yoga. By embracing diversity, promoting accessibility, and fostering a sense of belonging, yoga spaces can become environments where practitioners of all backgrounds can come together to experience unity, acceptance, and transformation on the mat. Inclusivity in yoga is not just about opening doors; it's about creating a space where everyone feels they truly belong.

Intention 2: Yoga for One increases yoga literacy

My second intention for the Yoga for One program is the promotion of yoga literacy. The term "yoga therapy" is inspired by the term "health literacy," which is well established in the public health promotion field to describe someone's ability to "know, understand, and apply" health information. I created the term "yoga literacy" to refer to a particular form of health literacy, focused on an individual's capacity to "know, understand, and apply" yoga philosophy, practices, and postures to improve personal health, wellness, and well-being.

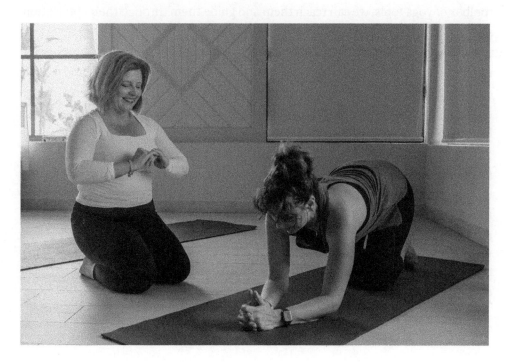

Most newcomers to yoga have low yoga literacy; they don't yet know the ways of the yoga world, nor do they understand how to modify the practice for their unique needs and preferences. When a newcomer starts yoga in a class setting, they often try to mimic other classmates and the instructor in the ways that they are performing the postures and practices, because they don't yet know how to adapt or modify them in ways that are best for their bodies. Newcomers may also push themselves in an effort to keep up with everyone else in the room. Instead of feeling the stress-reducing benefits of pulling over from their day to practice yoga with other yoga classmates, they may find themselves experiencing unexpected stress during the yoga class instead. A newcomer may also not realize that yoga is not just about postures.

On the other hand, in a one-on-one yoga setting, the newcomer can set healthy patterns for their minds and bodies early in the practice that can then continue with them over time. I have often found it ironic that newcomers to sports (such as golf) are encouraged to start out with one-on-one training with a professional so that they can build healthy patterns before playing on their own. I encourage yoga newcomers to take the same approach with yoga—so they can experience similar benefits, while feeling the support of a guide who is trained to help them.

Through one-on-one work with clients, we have the opportunity to help our clients to learn more about the many benefits that yoga has to offer them—yoga philosophy, practices, and postures. Once they become more familiar with this vast toolbox of yoga tools, we can teach them and guide them through their application, so they can better understand what yoga does and doesn't work well for them. Much like you would teach a young child to use scissors carefully, we can help them to understand why it is important that we use caution when practicing yoga so that we can stay safe and secure. Through improved yoga literacy, the client is less likely to become injured by a yoga practice that is not in their best interests, or traumatized by a yoga practice that is insensitive to their mental health needs.

Over time, the client's improved yoga literacy impacts their practice in other favorable ways. The client becomes more independent in yoga classes and community settings; they can make adjustments for themselves, whether or not the teacher notices they need a modification. They can apply yoga practices, postures, and philosophy throughout their day, whether or not they are in a class led by a teacher. They are able to practice yoga for themselves if and when they need to and want to. And the stress of being new to yoga diminishes because now yoga is a journey they know well enough to drive without directions.

Intention 3: Yoga for One establishes safe practice patterns

My third intention for the Yoga for One program is the establishment of safe yoga practice patterns. When I meet with new clients who have been referred by a doctor or trusted medical provider to "go try yoga," they often report that they are seeking yoga to help them with a particular life story plot twist, stress, or chronic illness. But what both they and their doctor may not realize is that their referral to yoga may unknowingly increase the odds of their patient (client) experiencing more harm than good. I say this with the utmost respect to yoga professionals who show up tirelessly in service to their classes and clients. I am speaking here to the communication problem that exists between medical providers and yoga professionals generally, which is no one's fault, but everyone's concern. Allow me to explain.

Most medical providers and most of the public are unaware that there are many styles of yoga. They may therefore unknowingly think that all yoga is created equal, without realizing that there are many styles of yoga that the patient (client) has to choose from, and that each style elicits a different effect. Their lack of knowledge about the many possibilities for yoga sets up a risky scenario in which the medical provider refers the patient to yoga and the patient tries a yoga practice that may or may not be in alignment with the medical provider's actual intentions.

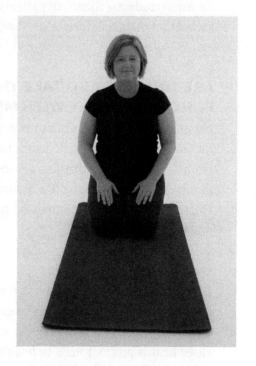

For example, the medical provider may refer a patient (client) to yoga as part of an overall aim to increase the patient's level of physical activity. However, if the patient decides to try a restorative yoga class, they may not realize that they would not be meeting the intention of the referral, because they would not be engaged in the same level of physical activity level that the medical provider intended. In a similar way, if the medical provider refers a patient (client) to yoga so that they can learn stress reduction techniques, but the patient finds themself in a hot vinyasa class taught in a "boot camp" style of cueing, the patient will not experience stress reduction. On the contrary, they would experience a heightened state of stress response in their sympathetic nervous system.

Further complicating this referral challenge is the challenge every teacher faces each time they set foot on their teaching mat. Because of the dynamics of a yoga class setting, yoga teachers do not usually have the time or space to check in with each student privately, to discuss the student's medical concern/s, personal preferences, and/or unique stress profile. And even in the rare cases when the yoga teacher is able to access this information and these insights, it can be difficult in a class setting to accommodate every individual need. Simply put, the more students there are, the more difficult it is for any teacher to tailor the practice in the specific and focused way that we can in a one-on-one yoga session.

Through the intentions of promoting inclusivity, increasing yoga literacy, and establishing safe practice patterns, the Yoga for One program ultimately aims to support humans (students, clients, or patients) in finding the yoga that works well for them in an experience that feels yogic (safe, supported, and compassionate).

ARE YOU READY TO TAKE THE YOGA FOR ONE JOURNEY WITH ME?

Now that you know more about why I wrote this book, and the intentions of a Yoga for One practice program, it is time to prepare for the journey we will take together. Before I outline what that journey looks like (by describing each chapter), I want to respectfully point out a few assumptions I am making for readers of this book. Please review these, and note whether or not they apply to you—and adapt your practice accordingly.

Our central assumptions

You are not new to yoga. This book is primarily written for yoga professionals (yoga coaches, yoga personal trainers, yoga teachers, and yoga therapists) who are open to learning a method I have developed for working with clients one-on-one. Other allied health professionals in healthcare and wellness settings who are already familiar with yoga may also find this book helpful for their one-on-one work with patients and clients. Because you are not new to yoga, we won't be spending time on what we might call "Yoga 101." You already know that the term "yoga" is derived from the Sanskrit word *yuj*, which means to yoke, or link together, and you know that the ultimate aim of yoga is to reach kaivalya (emancipation or ultimate freedom of the Self). You already have your own understanding of what yoga is for you, and you've found a way to reconcile the many definitions of yoga that are out there. You also have a general understanding of the 5000+ year history of yoga, and how it has changed so much over time. You know how yoga evolved from a practice of the privileged class in India to a practice for the common people, and how colonization, the growth of social media, and the reckoning on race have impacted it. You know that yoga is much more than a stretching regime, and that exciting findings are discovered every day in yoga research.

You have a daily sadhana (personal practice). As we learn in our yoga professional journey, yoga is an experiential science. Every day we meet ourselves on the mat (or wherever our sadhana takes us), we get to practice this science in the lab that is our mind–body–heart–spirit ecosystem. Through self-care, which I view more as self-leadership, we can generate the stamina we need to Serve others while protecting ourselves from the exhausting effects of burnout and compassion fatigue. Our daily sadhana also protects our students, clients, or patients from the negative impact of stress contagion—the phenomenon in which one human experiences a physiological reaction to another's stress response.

You are familiar with foundational yoga philosophy texts and the concepts and constructs found within them. Although you'll be able to navigate this book without having read these texts, your understanding of some of my conceptual references will be enhanced if you are familiar with them. You are ideally very familiar with the *Yoga Sutras of Patanjali,* and the brilliance of his distillation of the vast universe of yoga into his metaphor of the "8 limbs." You have ideally explored both the hero's journey in the *Bhagavad Gita* and the ancient truths about humanity of the *Upanishads,* and reflected on their meaning in your own life. You are familiar with the concepts of Purusha and Prakriti found within the *Samkhya Karika,* so you understand that one of the greatest power tools in our yoga toolbox is the ability to witness ourselves and our Self unconditionally in a divine state of acceptance and awe.

You endeavor to live the 8 limbs of yoga in your work and in your life. Because you are familiar with the *Yoga Sutras of Patanjali* (as noted above), you know that the "8 limbs" of yoga (aka Ashtanga Yoga) are a set of guiding principles and practices that form the foundation of classical yoga philosophy. You know and practice the five yamas in your daily interactions with the world, professionally and personally: ahimsa (non-violence), satya (truthfulness), asteya (non-stealing), brahmacharya (moderation), and aparigraha (non-possessiveness). You know and practice the personal observances, or niyamas, as part of your inner journey of spiritual discovery and self-purificiation: saucha (cleanliness), santosha (contentment), tapas (discipline), svadhyaya (self-study), and ishvarapranidhana (surrender to a higher power). You practice asanas (physical postures) to promote your physical health, strength, flexibility, and balance, and to prepare for meditation. You practice regulating and directing the control of your breath and your vitality through pranayama (practices of breath control). And you know how to apply the practices of pratyhara (withdrawal of the senses), dharana (concentration), and dhyana (focused meditation and deep absorption) to regulate your inner equilibrium and sense of overall harmony. You have experienced samadhi (enlightenment), or you are patiently practicing yoga as a means to its realization, because you know that yoga is a state of union with the divine in which a profound spiritual connection, inner peace, and experience of oneness are realized.

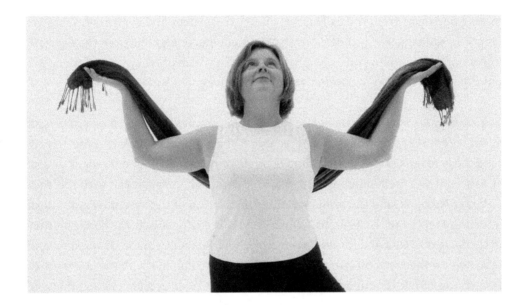

You do not share yoga philosophy, practices, or postures that you are not trained to share. As you may have learned in professional yoga education, our personal practice is not the same as our professional practice. It is important that we don't share practices that we haven't been trained to share. (Just because we practice them for ourselves doesn't mean we have been trained to safely share them with our students, clients, or patients.)

You know how to keep one professional hat on at a time, while staying within your unique scope of practice. Although you will see that I refer to you, the reader, as a yoga professional throughout this book, I first recognize that you have your own hat, or hats, that you wear professionally. You may be a yoga coach, yoga teacher, yoga personal trainer, yoga therapist, allied health professional integrating yoga into your work, or a trainer of yoga professionals. I want to reinforce here the importance of not wearing more than one hat at a time (so as not to confuse the student, client, or patient), and the importance of staying within the scope of your professional practice. I also want to remind you that this book is written for educational purposes only; none of this text or its lessons should be misconstrued as medical advice. As you learn the methodology and techniques I share in this book, I therefore ask that you stay grounded in your scope of practice, morally, ethically, and professionally.

You know the distinction between a yoga program and a plan of care. As the title implies, this book is designed to teach you how to co-create a yoga program for one human at a time, on and off the mat. Our approach to program co-creation is collaborative and not directive; we focus on ways that we can partner with our client in the act of co-creating the program rather than directing the client to follow a prescription or treatment plan. Although I invite licensed healthcare providers to explore how they can extract the process shared here into their work with their patients, I want to clarify for the reader that this is not our central intention. Put simply, we are not crossing the line of telling the human (student, client, or patient) what to do or not to do, as we would in a plan of care delivery. Rather, we are partnering with the human we are working with to assess where they are, envision where they want to be, and plan the trip between here and there together. In this way, we will ensure that we aren't diagnosing the human and/or prescribing yoga—practices that are out of scope for yoga professionals (including yoga coaches, yoga teachers, yoga trainers, yoga therapists, and trainers of these professionals). As the name implies, we are co-creating a program with our clients in an overall spirit of collaboration and partnership.

HOW DO WE GET STARTED?

Now that you know more about the Yoga for One journey in this book, it's time for us to get going on this journey. I am both personally and professionally glad you are here, to learn more about how you can co-create yoga programs one-on-one with clients. As the subtitle of the book implies, the process I will share with you aims to be inclusive and evidence-informed. We'll get to what I mean by these important terms—co-creation, inclusion, and evidence-informed—in Chapter 2.

In Chapter 3, we'll explore how you can prepare yourself and your business for the "company" of your clients. Although I am not an insurance agent, lawyer, or banker, and nor do I pretend to be, I will share with you what I wish someone had taught me when I started out about setting up your business for success, in a way that generates value for your clients. By the end of the chapter and its activities, you'll understand more about the basic business logistics that are important to consider as the foundation of your future work with clients.

In Chapter 4, we'll explore the pathway from marketing to monetization. Although most yoga professionals I know would rather not say the words "money" and "sales" out loud, I personally think it is time that we change that. We've got to be able to explain the value of our work to the clients who can afford to work with us and/or the investors and partners who can fund our work with the underserved (so they can sponsor clients who cannot afford our services). Marketing matters in both direct and third party payment models, which is why we have a whole chapter dedicated to the topic. In this chapter you'll learn my "9 Ps" for marketing—an expansion of the traditional "4 Ps."

In Chapter 5 we'll move into the actual work of program co-creation, with an entire chapter dedicated to meeting clients where they are through the practices of intake, interview, and assessment. This chapter walks you through my approach to the SOAP process (Subjective, Objective, Assessment, and Plan) using the science of sense-making. You'll also learn how you can use asanas as assessment tools, so you can learn more about your client's movement capability while also introducing them to foundational yoga postures.

Then, in Chapter 6, you'll learn how to apply what you have learned in the intake, interview, and assessment process in the design of an evidence-informed strategic program plan. In this chapter you'll learn how to use my logic model template to ensure that evaluation and assessment processes are embedded into your program plan design, to ensure that your program is aligned with your client's goals. You'll also learn more about the important distinction between impact, outcome, and output goals, and why they all matter for the client's buy-in to their program.

In Chapter 7 you'll learn how to address the priorities we established in Chapter 5, with particular sets of philosophy, postures, and practices based on the client's needs. You'll see how practices can be conceptually designed to bring balance to the client's social determinants of health, doshas, gunas, and koshas, in alignment with the goals set in their program plan.

CONCLUSION

As you can see, this journey is designed to support you in co-creating a yoga program for one person at a time. I look forward to sharing with you an approach that you can adapt to the needs of each person, so that we can prevent the practice of "cookie cutter" approaches that are one-size-fits-all. Instead, through our customized approach, we can help each student, client, or patient to experience yoga in a way that is uniquely tailored to their needs. We can feel confident knowing that we are co-creating a program with them that will support them in finding the yoga that is unique and authentic for them. And we can co-create an experience that is inclusive and evidence-informed, so that yoga can become more accessible for one...and all!

CHAPTER 2

Co-Creating Evidence-Informed Person-Centered Care

In this chapter you will learn how you can integrate both public health and health-care perspectives into the co-creation of a Yoga for One program. As someone who has worked in both contexts, I know they have unique points of view and standards, and I also know they have much in common.

WHY WE'RE TAKING AN EVIDENCE-INFORMED RATHER THAN EVIDENCE-BASED APPROACH

When I started sharing the title of this book with colleagues, clients, and students, one of the first questions they asked me was why I was using the term "evidence-informed" rather than "evidence-based." I therefore imagine that you, the reader, may be wondering the same thing.

In much the same way that many people use the terms "wellness" and "well-being" interchangeably, many use the terms "evidence-based" and "evidence-informed" interchangeably too. However, if you ask a wellness or well-being practitioner if there is a difference between wellness and well-being, they will answer with a resounding "yes." Wellness practitioners generally focus on how well we do our life (such as behavior change and lifestyle medicine), while well-being practitioners focus on how well we feel about our life (e.g., thriving, life satisfaction, and quality of life).

In a similar way, researchers, implementation scientists, and program developers have strong opinions about the use of the terms "evidence-based" vs. "evidence-informed." They all agree that the terms have different meanings; however, they disagree on which approach is preferred. Many advocates of evidence-based approaches believe these are preferable because they place great value on the scientific processes that have earned these approaches their evidence-based status.[4] From their perspective, the term "evidence-informed" implies that a program or protocol is in its initial pilot stages, or in the development process on the way to becoming evidence-based. These professionals may also believe that evidence-informed approaches are less scientifically mature than evidence-based approaches.

On the other hand, there are also many researchers and practitioners (including me) who place an entirely different meaning on the term "evidence-informed." According to Sullivan, Finlayson, and Moonaz (2017),[5] an evidence-informed practice approach is preferable in the practice of yoga therapy because it expands the focus on the best available evidence to also include provider expertise and client preferences. Their perspective is in alignment with the general trend in integrative health promotion to choose an evidence-informed approach over an evidence-based one. As noted by Chaturvedi *et al.* (2021),[6] an evidence-informed approach is more in keeping with the aims and practices of Ayurveda because it emphasizes the whole person.

As you can see in Figure 1, my approach to co-creating one-on-one yoga programs is evidence-informed. To simplify the process, I have streamlined the three perspectives that an evidence-informed approach offers into what I call the "3 Es": the client's lived *e*xperience; the best available *e*vidence in the research literature and in the "real life" of the client; and the *e*xpertise of the professional. In this choice of terms, I aim to enact the intentions and aims of evidence-informed practice by valuing the best available evidence (otherwise known as the current evidence basis); the expertise of the facilitator and their practice field; and the client's lived experience. This type of contextualization reduces the likelihood of bias that can more easily occur when only one point of view is offered: "Blending knowledge from different sources is an inclusive and useful approach because knowledge is personal, context driven and evolving. This type of approach also allows for innovation and adaptation based on factors and context at individual, organizational and service levels, while reducing biases."[7]

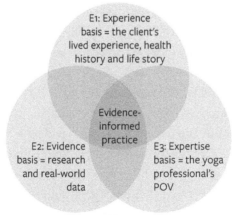

Note: POV = point of view

FIGURE 1: YOGA FOR ONE EVIDENCE-INFORMED 3 ES MODEL

EVIDENCE-BASED OR EVIDENCE-INFORMED?

As we have seen, the terms "evidence-based" and "evidence-informed" sound similar, but they differ in their scope and application. Let's explore their meaning.

Evidence-based practice (EBP):

- *Origin:* EBP originated in the medical field, with the aim of making clinical decisions based on the best available, current, scientific evidence.

- *Definition:* The integration of clinical expertise, patient values and preferences, and the best research evidence into the decision-making process for patient care.

- *Components:*

  - *Clinical expertise:* Knowledge and skills of the healthcare professional.
  - *Patient preferences and values:* Each patient is unique and has their own preferences, concerns, and expectations.
  - *Best research evidence:* Rigorous research, typically from randomized controlled trials or systematic reviews.
  - *Focus:* The emphasis is often on quantitative research, especially randomized controlled trials, as these are considered the "gold standard" in determining the effectiveness of treatments.
  - *Limitation:* Can sometimes be viewed as rigid due to its strong emphasis on research evidence, potentially neglecting clinician experience or patient preferences.

Evidence-informed practice (EIP):

- *Origin:* EIP evolved from EBP to address the concerns that evidence-based practice might be too narrow in its approach, especially in fields outside of medicine.

- *Definition:* An approach that seeks to integrate the best available evidence with professional expertise, while considering the unique characteristics, preferences, and lived experiences of the client or population being served.

- *Components:*

  - *Professional expertise:* Skills, knowledge, and judgment acquired through education and experience.
  - *Client characteristics, culture, and preferences:* Recognizing the diverse backgrounds and needs of individuals or populations.

- *Best available evidence:* While this includes rigorous research, it also values other forms of evidence such as case studies, qualitative research, and experiential knowledge.
- *Focus:* Embraces a broader spectrum of evidence, including both quantitative and qualitative research. Recognizes that high-quality randomized controlled trials might not be available or applicable for all situations.
- *Flexibility:* Offers a more holistic and flexible approach. Recognizes that decisions are often made in contexts where perfect evidence isn't available, and other factors must be considered.

Both EBP and EIP emphasize the importance of evidence in guiding practice. EBP takes a mostly empirical approach, emphasizing objectivity and aiming for rigor. EIP takes a mostly formative approach, and adopts a more inclusive and flexible stance. EIP values a wider range of evidence types and emphasizes the importance of context, professional judgment, and individual or population characteristics in decision-making. Our Yoga for One approach is evidence-informed, in keeping with our aim to stay client-centered.

HEALTHCARE AND PUBLIC HEALTH POINTS OF VIEW

Both healthcare and public health play crucial roles in promoting well-being and preventing disease, but they approach the promotion of health, wellness, and well-being from different points of view. When co-creating client-centered one-on-one yoga programs, we encourage you to integrate the best of both approaches while staying within your unique scope of practice.

Generally speaking, yoga teachers focus on a public health approach, because they focus on education and prevention. Meanwhile, yoga therapists and allied health professionals integrate both healthcare and public health approaches based on the needs of their clients. Let's explore how these two points of view are both similar and yet different.

Healthcare point of view

- *Individual focus:* A healthcare approach focuses on medicine—generally, the individualized treatment of one person at a time. A healthcare approach to yoga is in keeping with the practice of yoga therapy, in which the certified yoga therapist tailors sessions to the specific needs, conditions, or goals of the individual client.[8]

- *Diagnosis and treatment:* Although most yoga professionals are not professionally permitted to diagnose or prescribe yoga, because it is not within their scope of practice, yoga can be offered as a complementary practice to clients with a specific condition. In some cases, the yoga program can be tailored to address the stress of the client's given illness, while in other cases it can be tailored to support the client with the symptoms of the illness or the side effects of medications.

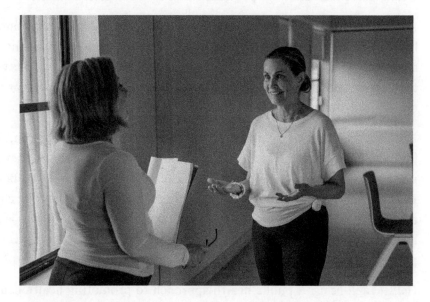

- *Therapeutic context:* Yoga programs can be recommended by a doctor or other allied health professional (such as a physical therapist or mental health professional) as part of an individual's broader therapeutic or rehabilitation regimen.

- *Risk management:* Through a tailored yoga program, the yoga professional can support the client in ensuring that certain poses or practices do not exacerbate existing conditions. Contraindications based on individual health status can be carefully considered.

- *Measurable outcomes:* In our Yoga for One program approach, we integrate planning and evaluation into the program design process (as noted later, in Chapter 6). This approach means that we aim to assess and measure program outcomes, so that we can track the client's progress towards their specific goals, such as reductions in pain, increased range of motion, or improved cardiovascular measures.

Public health point of view

- *Population health:* A public health point of view places importance on the social determinants of health, and explores how they impact individuals, communities, regions, and cultures. In a one-on-one yoga program, we can take this approach by recognizing that the individual is impacted by these social determinants of health. In Chapter 7, we will explore strategies for attuning a one-on-one yoga program based on these determinants.

- *Prevention:* A public health point of view considers the full continuum of health outcomes, from prevention to treatment. By taking a public health approach, we can design one-on-one yoga programs that support clients with their current health concerns while also aiming to help them to prevent new ones from occurring.

- *Education and awareness:* A public health point of view values education, aiming to build the health literacy of the individual or population so that they can make more informed and strategic choices for their health and well-being. In a one-on-one yoga program, we can aim to go beyond leading the client through certain practices to also educate them on what is and what is not beneficial for their unique health situation (based on the latest evidence and public health guidance).

- *Holistic well-being:* A public health approach to promoting health can be holistic, and this is in alignment with yoga's holistic point of view. Instead of focusing narrowly on specific ailments, there is a broader emphasis on overall well-being, including mental, emotional, and social health.

- *Community linkages:* A public health-oriented yoga professional can connect their one-on-one clients with community resources or recommend group classes, seeing the value in community engagement and social connection as part of health. Some yoga professionals (including me) also offer their one-on-one clients the opportunity to meet to build peer and community support (outside the one-on-one session).

As you can see, while both approaches value the health benefits of yoga for the individual client, a *healthcare point of view* tends to be more individualistic, focusing on specific ailments and conditions. A *public health point of view* recognizes the individual within the context of their community and environment, emphasizing prevention, holistic well-being, and the broader social determinants of health. A healthcare point of view is more in alignment with a yoga therapy practice, while a public health point of view is more in alignment with the field of yoga education (teaching). Because yoga therapists begin as yoga teachers (as part of their professional pathway), they have the professional capacity to integrate both approaches into the co-creation of one-on-one yoga programs.

Because the primary audience for this book is yoga teachers, we will take a primarily public health approach throughout this journey. However, you (as the reader) are encouraged to reflect on which approach is best aligned with your professional practice.

WHAT IS THE SOCIO-ECOLOGICAL MODEL?

In public health practice, we have a model that helps us to conceptualize, understand, and apply the ripple effect of impact that an intervention makes. This model is called the "socio-ecological model" (see Figure 2).[9] We use this model to make decisions on where we will focus our efforts in the design of a public health intervention. The model assumes that no matter where we focus our efforts for an intervention, it will create a ripple effect to the other levels. For example, if we design an intervention for parents of students in a school setting, we know that there will be a ripple effect of impact to the students (as their parents' children), the faculty and staff of the school (through their school-based interactions), and the community at large (because the parents are part of, and interact with, the community).

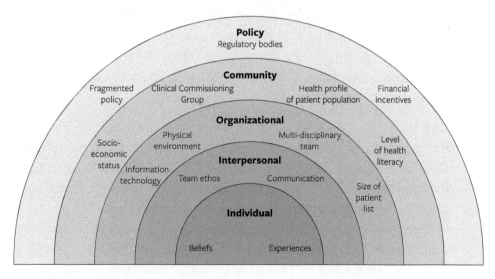

FIGURE 2: SOCIO-ECOLOGICAL FRAMEWORK SHOWING THE
INFLUENCES ON PATIENT SAFETY IN PRIMARY CARE[10]

Let's explore what we mean by each level, and how they each offer their own unique benefits for creating a healthy ripple effect across all the levels, to advance population health and well-being.

How does the socio-ecological model explain the health ripple effect?

- *Individual level:* At the core of this model are the individual's personal characteristics, behaviors, and genetics, which are influenced by their outer contexts (other levels) as well as their intrapersonal engagement (within themselves). Yoga offers a wide range of asanas (physical postures), pranayama (breath control), and meditation practices to cultivate the practitioner's optimization at this level, promoting self-awareness, mindfulness, and healthier choices.

- *Interpersonal level:* Moving outward in the model, the interpersonal level illustrates the influence of relationships on the individual, and the impact of social support and peer norms on personal (individual) health, wellness, and well-being. Yoga encourages the individual to practice compassion, empathy, and ahimsa (non-violence) in their engagement with others. Yoga practice with family and friends can support healthier relationships, by providing a forum for practicing trust and communication.

- *Organizational level:* The organizational level accounts for the physical environment and/or team setting within which a Yoga for One program is delivered. For example, a client may work with a yoga professional in a hospital setting, in a yoga studio, or online through a privacy-secure telehealth portal. The service delivery of a Yoga for One program may be a stand-alone with each client, or may be part of an overarching approach to care delivered in an integrative health setting.

- *Community level:* This level illustrates how the neighborhoods we live in and the organizations we operate in impact us interpersonally (in our relationships), intrapersonally (within ourselves), and societally. The community level also explores how the built environment, access to resources, and community cohesion affect the health of community populations—whether they are neighborhood- or online-based. Yoga studios and wellness centers often serve as hubs for building community among yoga practitioners, providing them with a safe space for practice and a refuge from their daily challenges while also promoting healthy behaviors and social support. Yoga retreats and other community events create spaces for shared experiences that enhance the feeling of belonging to a community, which helps to reduce isolation and enhance well-being.

- *Policy level:* The outermost layer of the socio-ecological model encompasses the broader societal, cultural, and political contexts that impact communities, relationships, and individuals. This level examines economic systems, government policies, and cultural norms, recognizing their profound impact on health, with an emphasis on the health disparities that can arise between individuals and populations based on environmental, cultural, and political factors. We can bring yoga practice and the study of yoga philosophy to this level when we promote ethical principles (yamas and niyamas) and encourage individuals to promote social justice, equality, and compassion. Yoga communities can also engage in social activism and charitable activities, which serve the communities, families, and individuals that are underserved and in need of support.

HOW CAN WE REDUCE HEALTH DISPARITIES AND ADVANCE HEALTH EQUITY?

In the public health practice field, much of our work aims to reduce health disparities, at all levels of the socio-ecological model. *Health disparities*, also known as *health inequities*, refers to the systemic differences in health outcomes between different groups or populations. These can be seen in rates of diseases, disabilities, and overall mortality. For example, some groups may experience higher rates of chronic diseases like diabetes, heart disease, or cancer, leading to poorer health outcomes.

The following factors have been identified as some of the fundamental areas to address to reduce health disparities while promoting health equity:

- *Age-related disparities:* Health disparities can vary by age, with certain age groups, such as children, seniors, and adolescents, experiencing unique health challenges.

- *Racial and ethnic disparities:* Racial and minority ethnic groups, in many countries, often experience higher rates of health disparities compared to the majority population. These can be due to a combination of social, economic, and systemic factors.

- *Gender and identity disparities:* Many people have gender identities that do not fit within the cisgender (binary) categories of "male" and "female." Health disparities can occur within each gender or identity group, and across multiple gender identities.

- *Geographic disparities:* Rural and urban areas may experience different levels of healthcare access and quality, leading to health disparities across geographic regions.

- *Access and quality of healthcare:* Differences in access to healthcare services can contribute to health disparities. Some individuals or communities may need more access to primary care, specialists, or preventive services, leading to delayed or inadequate healthcare. Some individuals may delay seeking care due to barriers such as cost, transportation, or cultural factors. Certain groups may receive healthcare treatment differently than other groups, causing disparities in the appropriateness of treatment, patient–provider communication, and adherence to clinical guidelines.

- *Health behaviors:* Disparities can be linked to variations in health behaviors such as smoking, diet, physical activity, and substance misuse. These behaviors can impact the risk of developing certain health conditions.

Addressing health disparities is a critical public health and societal goal that involves efforts to reduce and ultimately eliminate these unjust differences in health outcomes. Health equity will be achieved when all individuals have the same opportunities to achieve their best possible health regardless of their background or circumstances. Although we know there is much work to be done to reduce health disparities and realize a global state of health equity, I also believe that we can do our part to advance health equities and to reduce health disparities by taking an inclusive and evidence-informed approach to the co-creation of one-on-one yoga programs.

A CLOSER LOOK AT THE SOCIAL DETERMINANTS OF HEALTH

As we have seen, the *social determinants of health* (SDOH) are the conditions in which people are born, grow, live, work, and age. These factors are shaped by social, economic, and political forces that have a profound influence on an individual's health and quality of life, and whether or not they will experience the negative consequences of health disparities. Although different public health practitioners and scholars disagree on the specific list of the social determinants of health, the following are the most widely accepted:

- *Economic stability:* Income level and regularity are closely linked to health outcomes. Poverty and income inequality can result in limited access to nutritious food, safe housing, and quality healthcare.

- *Education access:* Education is a powerful determinant of health. People with higher levels of education are able to secure occupations that provide them with safer living conditions and better access to healthcare. They are also more likely to have received health education during their school years, which increases the likelihood that they are making healthier choices and experiencing improved well-being.

- *Social and community context:* Social factors like social support, discrimination, and community cohesion shape health outcomes. Strong social connections and supportive relationships are protective factors for health. Isolation and lack of social support can lead to adverse health effects.

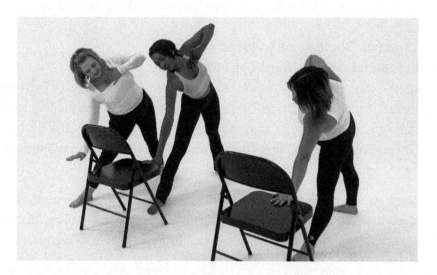

- *Access to healthcare:* Affordable and accessible healthcare services are crucial for maintaining good health. Barriers to healthcare access, such as lack of health insurance or geographic distance, can lead to health disparities.

- *Neighborhood and built environment:* The built environment, including access to safe housing, clean air and water, and recreational spaces, significantly influences health.

- *Healthy food access:* Not everyone has access to healthy foods. A food desert is an area, typically in urban or rural settings, where there is limited access to affordable and nutritious food. These areas are often characterized by the absence of grocery stores, farmers' markets, and other sources of fresh and healthy food options. People living in food deserts may rely heavily on convenience stores or fast food outlets for their meals, which tend to offer more processed and less nutritious options. Food deserts can contribute to health disparities and issues such as malnutrition, obesity, and chronic diseases, as residents may have difficulty accessing the ingredients needed for a balanced diet.

- *Employment and working conditions:* Job security, work-related stress, and occupational hazards can impact physical and mental health. Unemployment and underemployment can lead to financial instability and negative health outcomes, while optimal employment can promote purpose, well-being, and what yogis and yoginis refer to as the "realization of one's dharma."

- *Cultural and social engagement:* Cultural beliefs and societal norms can impact health behaviors, including diet, exercise, and seeking medical care.

How Yoga for One can be tailored for the person's social determinants of health

Although the co-creation of a Yoga for One program can't change an individual's social determinants of health, we can tailor a program to the challenges that are associated with them as part of an overarching effort to reduce health disparities. The following are a few examples of how we can customize a Yoga for One program based on the social determinants of health:

- *Stress reduction:* Tailoring yoga techniques for an individual's needs can help them to manage the stress related to their social determinants of health, such as economic hardship, limited access to healthcare, or gender identity disparities.

- *Mind–body connection:* The Yoga for One co-creation process emphasizes the mind–body–heart–spirit connection, encouraging the individual to be more in tune with their body and emotions. This can lead to better self-awareness and improved decision-making regarding their health behaviors, which can help them to offset the challenges of their health disparities with prevention-based solutions.

- *Cultivating resilience:* Through the tailored delivery of a Yoga for One program, a yoga professional can support the individual in developing their emotional resilience and coping skills, which can be particularly valuable for individuals facing adversity.

- *Social support:* Through the one-on-one support of a Yoga for One provider, an individual can experience the social support of a partner dedicated to helping them in achieving their health and well-being goals. This experience can counter feelings of isolation and provide a sense of belonging.

- *Accessible practices:* The Yoga for One process aims to meet the physical, emotional, and financial needs of clients, thereby making it accessible to a broad range of individuals.

- *Education and awareness:* Through the Yoga for One co-creation process, yoga professionals educate clients about the impact of the social determinants on their health. This process, in turn, helps the student, client, or patient to better navigate healthcare systems and resources effectively, and improves their yoga literacy (health literacy as applied to the study of yoga philosophy and the sadhana of yoga postures and practices).

A CLOSER LOOK AT PERSON-CENTERED CARE

Person-centered care is an approach to healthcare endorsed by the World Health Organization (WHO). Although it is an approach that is often familiar to professionals in the healthcare system, it has been my experience that the term is often new to yoga professionals. At first glance, "person-centered" seems simple and relatively straightforward—put the client at the center of their care experience. However, there is much more to the story of person-centered care when we consider how we can put this concept into actual practice.

The first challenge that we can easily find in putting a person-centered care approach into practice is found in the name we use to refer to it. For example, in the biomedical healthcare practice field, *patient-centered care* is used, while in integrative health and yoga practice fields, *client-centered care* is used. Although the terms are different in these different contexts, they are both referring to the notion that the client is at the center.

These different terms also reveal some underlying assumptions that are found in biomedical healthcare vs. integrative health contexts. The term "patient" evolved in the 14th century, and is derived from the Latin word *patiens*, meaning "to suffer" or "to endure." There is an implication with the use of the term "patient" that the individual experiencing disease, ailment, or injury is suffering from the disease problem. The biomedical approach focuses on the delivery of healthcare to address the patient's pathology/ies as the way to reduce suffering.

In contrast to this biomedical approach is the integrative health approach to

person-centered care. In the integrative health practice field (in which yoga professional practice fields reside), the person receiving care is referred to as a "client,"
or "health consumer." This term reveals an underlying assumption that the person
receiving care is an active participant in their care plan. They are seen less as someone who is suffering (patient) who must be treated with directives placed on them,
and more as someone who has the power to engage actively in their care process,
and to choose which treatments, behaviors, and/or experiences are in alignment
with their holistic needs.

In the yoga practice field, the term "client" is generally used to refer to the
person receiving care—showing the field's alignment with other integrative health
fields. I believe we must use caution when we use this term in any one-on-one yoga
program co-creation. It can inaccurately imply that the person receiving care is
paying for integrative healthcare services, when, in fact, other payment models can
be established. For example, a third party grantor or organization may sponsor a
one-on-one yoga program for an individual, meaning that the person receiving care
is not a client in the commercial sense of the term.

The five principles of person-centered care

Although there are many perspectives on best practices in the delivery of
person-centered care, I have found through my research and my work in the practice
field that there are five key principles in the delivery of person-centered care. Let's
explore them now:

- *Whole person and integrative health:* The person-centered care approach places
  the person receiving healthcare at the center of a wheel of allied health providers. This approach acknowledges that each individual is multi-dimensional,
  with a unique set of physical, mental, emotional, and social needs. As a result,
  person-centered care aims to meet each individual in their own unique needs,
  while recognizing that each person may respond to care differently too.

- *Continuity and coordination of care:* Person-centered care emphasizes the
  importance of continuity and coordination of care across different healthcare
  settings and providers. It aims to ensure that individuals receive seamless
  and well-coordinated care, with clear communication and smooth transitions
  between healthcare professionals.

- *Empathy and compassion:* Empathy and compassion are essential components of person-centered care. Healthcare and wellness providers strive to
  understand and empathize with the emotions, fears, and concerns of their

patients and clients, creating a compassionate and supportive environment that enhances their overall care experience. In this person-centered care approach, the person receiving care's experience of care becomes as important as the care itself.

- *Collaboration and relationships:* Person-centered care promotes collaboration between healthcare providers and those they are caring for (aka the patients). It recognizes that those receiving care have unique insights into their own lived experiences and values, and encourages them to openly and honestly communicate with their care team about them, so that their plan of care can be adjusted accordingly. The person-centered care approach emphasizes long-term relationships between the person receiving care and their team of allied health providers (sometimes referred to as their *ring of care*).

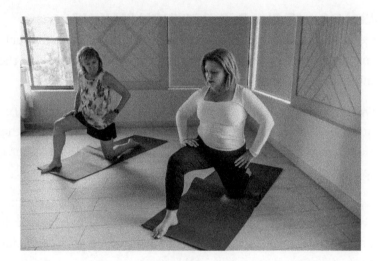

- *Autonomy in shared decision-making:* In the person-centered care approach, the person receiving care and their allied health team engage in shared decision-making. As this implies, shared decision-making is a collaborative approach to healthcare in which those receiving care (patients) and healthcare providers work together to make informed decisions about the care plan, taking into account the patient's values, preferences, and the best available evidence.

The benefits of person-centered care

When person-centered care is implemented in the way it is intended—and the client feels supported by the entire care team—multiple benefits are achieved. The four primary benefits of person-centered care are shown in Table 1:

Table 1: Person-centered care outcomes

Improved health outcomes	When clients feel empowered and engaged, they are more likely to adhere to treatment plans, manage chronic conditions effectively, and experience better overall health
Improved client (patient) satisfaction	As clients feel heard, respected, and actively involved in their care decisions, they are more likely to adhere to their care plan, and therefore become more satisfied with their care
Increased healthcare efficiency	Through coordination and continuity of care, person-centered care can reduce unnecessary healthcare utilization and other inefficiencies, resulting in cost savings (resources and personnel)
Improved quality of life	Clients who feel supported on their care journey have higher well-being and less experience of illness (even when managing disease)

A CLOSER LOOK AT SHARED DECISION MAKING

Through the shared decision-making process, the client maintains the central "starring role" in this decision-making process, and they engage actively in the design, delivery, and evaluation of their care in the following ways:

- *Information sharing*: Healthcare providers share the client's medical condition, treatment options, risks, benefits, and potential outcomes with them. They present this information in a clear and understandable manner, which is adapted to the client's health literacy and health numeracy level.

- *Patient's values and preferences*: Clients are encouraged to express their values, preferences, and goals related to their healthcare. This may include discussing what matters most to them in terms of quality of life, treatment side effects, spiritual beliefs, and other personal factors.

- *Discussion of options*: Clients and medical providers discuss the available treatment or care options, including the pros and cons of each. This includes exploring alternative treatments or the option of not pursuing treatment if appropriate.

- *Decision support*: Decision aids, such as written materials, videos, or decision support tools, may be used to help clients better understand their options and the potential outcomes associated with each choice.

- *Deliberation*: Clients are given time to consider their options, consult with loved ones if desired, and reflect on what choice aligns best with their values and preferences.

- *Collaboration:* The final decision is made collaboratively between the client and the healthcare provider. This decision should respect the client's autonomy and choices.

- *Follow-up and re-evaluation:* After a healthcare decision is made, ongoing communication between the client and medical provider is essential regarding the decision and its impact. This process allows for adjustments to the care plan if needed, and ensures that the client's preferences are respected throughout the treatment process.

Communication strategies for shared decision-making

In the process of shared decision-making, the healthcare provider and the client progress through three phases (components) of shared decision-making:[11]

- *Choice talk:* The client has the opportunity to choose the key components of their care plan. In co-creation of a one-on-one yoga program, the client would be able to choose whether or not their program focuses on their practice of yoga on the mat and/or their practice of lifestyle medicine off the mat. The client will also be able to choose postures or other practices of yoga based on their preferences. In this way, the client is making active choices throughout the practice, rather than receiving postures that have been pre-determined by others.

- *Option talk:* The client is also educated on the "why" (or potential value) behind the choices they are being offered. This serves to equip them with additional insights and information that informs their decision-making process. For example, instead of being asked to make a choice based on how they feel (choice talk), they are also taught why two choices could be helpful to them. The client can then make a choice not only on their preferences, but also based on their best interests.

- *Decision talk:* During this phase in the shared decision-making process, clients are encouraged to reflect on how each option is personally meaningful to them. Here the client is able to reflect on the potential impact each choice can make on their yoga practice and their life, and they are encouraged to connect intuitively to the meaning-making of each practice as it relates to their life story.

▦ HOW WE MAKE IT ALL HAPPEN: THE CO-CREATION PROCESS

Co-creation is a collaborative process in which individuals work together to create value, solutions, or outcomes. Through the process of co-creation, a collective wisdom is generated that would not otherwise be possible without collaboration. By involving everyone in the process of shared decision-making, co-creation promotes a more inclusive, participatory, and democratic approach to innovation, problem solving, and service delivery. As individuals bring their unique perspectives, assumptions, and cultural backgrounds into the process of co-creation, the process of shared decision-making transforms into shared meaning and understanding. Better solutions are generated because people have the opportunity to hear from, and listen to, everyone's perspectives.

Co-creation goes beyond traditional teaching methods by fostering a dynamic collaboration between the instructor and the participant. It shifts the paradigm from a one-size-fits-all approach to one that is tailored, deeply engaged, and rooted in mutual understanding and shared objectives. By integrating co-creation, yoga professionals ensure that each session not only addresses the physical aspects of the practice, but also resonates with the individual's emotional, mental, and spiritual journey.

The following components elucidate the essence and imperative nature of co-creation:

- *Collaborative:* The co-creation process requires collaboration between, and active participation from, different stakeholders, fostering a stronger sense of ownership and engagement among participants. In much the same way, the Yoga for One approach relies on active collaboration between the program facilitator and the participant so that all voices are heard and honored.

- *Value-oriented:* Co-creation focuses on generating value by producing outcomes that are meaningful to the program's intended participants and beneficiaries. The Yoga for One approach prioritizes the importance of value generation, which we will explore further in Chapters 3 and 4.

- *Human-centered design:* The co-creation process is closely related to the concept of human-centered design, which prioritizes the "user's experience" (otherwise known as the program participant's experience). By collaborating with end users to co-create user-friendly and user-driven solutions, a Yoga for One program team can ensure that a program is functional, enjoyable, and relevant.

- *Iterative process:* Co-creation follows an iterative process, where ideas, prototypes, or solutions are continuously refined based on feedback and input from participants. This flexibility allows for improvements and adjustments along the way. Businesses take this approach when they involve customers in the co-design of products, services, and processes so that they can better meet customer expectations. In the same way, the Yoga for One program approach is also iterative.

The value proposition for co-creation

In the delivery of one-on-one yoga programs, co-creation shows up as a way of operating and being with our clients. In this chapter, we have explored the importance of taking an evidence-informed approach from both the healthcare and public health points of view. How we actually do that is through the process of co-creation. Using co-creation as your "way of being and operating" with clients offers you and your clients the following value proposition (benefits):

- *Empowerment and self-awareness:* Co-creation empowers those receiving care by involving them in decision-making and encouraging active participation. This process cultivates self-awareness, as participants develop a deeper understanding of their own needs, preferences, and capabilities. Empowered individuals are more likely to take ownership of their well-being and actively engage in the entire yoga practice program design and evaluation process.

- *Enhanced mind–body connection:* Co-creation invites those receiving care to feel supported in listening to and honoring their bodies, reflecting on these experiences, and discussing them to the degree to which they are comfortable. By actively participating in the shared decision-making process, participants become more attuned to their own physical and emotional sensations, leading to a stronger mind–body connection. This enhanced awareness allows individuals to adapt the practice to their unique needs and optimize its benefits.

- *Increased engagement and enjoyment:* When those receiving care are actively involved in shaping their yoga practice, they experience a greater sense of engagement and enjoyment. Co-creation fosters a positive and inclusive environment, where participants feel valued and heard. This positive experience can deepen their commitment to regular practice and enhance the overall enjoyment of the yoga experience.

- *Personalized and targeted practice:* Co-creation in yoga enables personalized and targeted practices that address individual needs and goals. By incorporating the preferences, intentions, and feedback of those receiving care, yoga therapists, yoga mentors, and yoga teachers can tailor the practice to focus on specific areas of well-being, such as stress reduction, flexibility, or mindfulness. This customization enhances the effectiveness and relevance of the practice for each participant.

The key components of co-creation

Now that you are familiar with the principles of co-creation, it is time to explore how we can actually make the co-creation process happen. Although every co-creation effort is different, there are several key components in the process:

- *Establish a safe and inclusive environment*: Creating a safe and inclusive environment is crucial for co-creation. When the yoga professional cultivates an atmosphere of trust, respect, and non-judgment, those receiving care feel comfortable expressing their needs and preferences.

- *Open communication and active listening*: Effective communication and active listening are essential for co-creation. When a yoga professional encourages participants to openly communicate their expectations, limitations, preferences, and feedback, they can aim to actively listen, acknowledge what they have heard, and incorporate learned insights into the practice program.

- *Individual assessments and goal setting*: Prior to starting a yoga practice, individual assessments can help determine the client's specific needs and goals, and any physical or emotional considerations. Based on these assessments, co-creation can occur through collaborative goal setting, tailoring the practice to meet individual objectives.

- *Adaptations and modifications*: Co-creation can be a way to approach modifications and adaptations for the practice. Through ongoing communication (both verbal and non-verbal) the yoga professional can adapt and modify the practice in order to accommodate the client's preferences, abilities, and limitations. This process may involve providing variations of poses, using props, or offering different styles of yoga.

A Samkhya philosophy perspective on co-creation

As we have learned, co-creation is a process of collaboration that drives to client-centered outcomes. When yoga professionals and program participants engage in the co-creation process of a yoga program, they are bringing what has previously not been manifested into material (programmatic) form. There is a natural act of witnessing that occurs in this process: the yoga professional (ideally) holds space for and witnesses the client in their true nature. Interestingly this process of manifestation aligns well with the Samkhya philosophy principles of Purusha and Prakriti:

- *Purusha* is the concept of the eternal, unchanging, and transcendent consciousness or spirit. In the context of co-creation, Purusha represents the pure, unmanifested potential and the essence of existence. In the context of co-creation, Purusha can be seen as the source of inspiration, creativity, and higher consciousness that individuals tap into during collaborative processes. Here, Purusha can also represent the deeper wisdom and guidance that individuals access to contribute their unique insights and ideas. Purusha inspires individuals to connect with their inner selves, and brings forth their authentic contributions in the co-creation process.

- *Prakriti* refers to the manifest, material nature of the universe, including the physical world, matter, energy, and the diversity of forms. In the context of co-creation, Prakriti represents the dynamic and diverse nature of the individuals, ideas, and perspectives involved in the collaborative process. Like the interplay of the gunas, co-creation involves the interaction of different qualities, perspectives, and energies. The diverse contributions and interactions in co-creation reflect the ever-changing nature of Prakriti. The process of co-creation can feel at times dynamic (sattvic), at other times turbulent (rajasic), and at other times slow (tamasic)—just like Prakriti (our true nature) can experience these qualities (or movements) of matter.

In the process of co-creation, it is as though we, as the yoga professional, are playing the role of Purusha—we hold the client in positive regard and see them and their potentiality (the true nature of Prakriti) in a way that they cannot see. The client is seeking to discover their true inner nature of Prakriti by leaving their state of imbalance (Vikriti).

As Purusha and Prakriti witness each other, co-creation begins. An interplay between the transcendent and the material, the unmanifested and the manifested occurs organically through the practice and process of co-creation.

A Tantra philosophy perspective on co-creation

In the co-creation of a one-on-one yoga program, we can also find inspiration from the Tantra tradition. As a grass-roots movement, in which yoga philosophy and practices moved out of the esoteric settings of the privileged class and into the daily practices of the working class, the Tantra movement symbolically took yoga out of its own head and brought it down into the experience of the body. Through

Tantra, the modern-day notion that yoga can be an embodiment of ideals and an experiential science emerged.

The Tantra movement was inspired greatly by Shiva and Shakti (divine masculine and feminine) power that was originally illuminated in the *Vedas*. Shakti, with her creative energy and power, gives rise to the diverse forms and experiences within the universe. She is comprised of three functions of creative action—namely kriya (creative action), iccha (creative will), and jnana (creative wisdom). Shiva, with his transcendent awareness, holds the space for the unfolding of creation, and provides the underlying stability needed to keep the union in place. Together, Shakti and Shiva dance together in a harmonious act of co-creation.[12]

When we are co-creating a yoga program for one-on-one clients, we are symbolically serving in the Shiva role: we are holding space for the unfolding of creation with an underlying stability needed for the co-creation to occur. We can support the client in finding their own Shakti within—their place of creative energy, creative will, and creative wisdom. The client has the full capacity to engage in this work independently; they have all of the answers within. But it is through the connection we make with them in our transcendent awareness that we provide the space for co-creation to occur. Here, the alchemy of Shiva and Shakti connect in primordial fashion, manifesting something out of nothing. This process isn't sexual (as Tantra is often mistaken to be), but it is unifying and fortifying. Here we move beyond notions of dualism and find the Yoga for One.

HOW YOU CAN BEGIN "DOING" CO-CREATION USING THE "COACH" FRAMEWORK

As an advocate for co-creation in yoga one-on-one delivery, yoga professionals often ask me how they can go about the day-to-day work (and play) of enacting the co-creation process. It has been my lived experience that most yoga professionals are on board with the idea of co-creation; however, it is the putting it into practice that becomes difficult.

For this reason, I developed a strategy framework called "C-O-A-C-H," which offers a concise strategy for co-creation in the delivery of a one-on-one yoga program (and it is also transportable to other one-on-one service delivery). I chose the particular word COACH as the acronym because it is inspired by the professional practice of coaching. Whether or not you are formally trained as a coach, you can use this framework as a checklist for components with the co-creation process. Let's review each letter and see how you can apply this framework to foster healing presence with your clients.

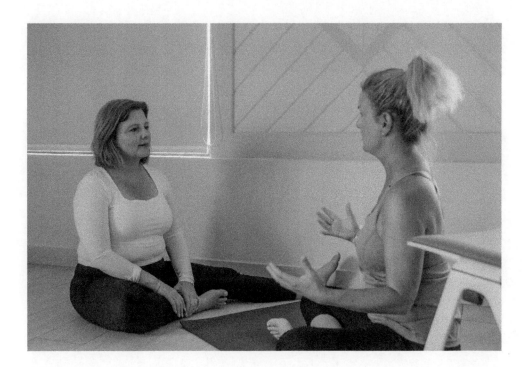

C stands for centering ourselves before we hold space for the client. If we are going to have the stamina needed to show up fully for the co-creation process with our clients, we need to be in a centered state of mind ourselves. A commitment to our personal practice (sadhana) is therefore an imperative for our own well-being as well as for our work.

O stands for opening up the conversation. In our soundbite world, we often think we have to be short and sweet. But there is also value in encouraging the client to expand their thinking, and to literally think out loud. Oftentimes, as they open up in their answers to open (vs. closed) questions, they find answers that they have within. So let's give them space for that.

A is for asking and not telling. Here we acknowledge that it is important to ask the client to reflect on what they do and don't care about, and what they do and don't want. It's important that we use the power of facilitation here to ask them questions that invite their self-reflection and self-inquiry, without telling them what to do, think, or feel. In this way we are respecting their life story and also engaging in person-centered care.

C stands for choices, which is a key ingredient in the science of shared decision-making and the process of co-creation. As we spend more time asking the client about their values, preferences, needs, and goals (than we do telling the client what we feel they should or shouldn't be doing), we can empower them to have both agency and autonomy in their program design. Through the process of shared decision-making, we facilitate the client's choice-making process, while providing the client with information and education when they need it so that they can make the choices that are best for them. As we encourage the client to exercise their autonomy in making their own choices, rather than "telling them what to do and when," we increase the likelihood that the client will like the program and stay motivated to complete it because they played an active role in its creation.

H is for holding our client in positive regard, holding space for them with compassion, and enacting healing presence. Here we do all that we can to support the client with non-judgmental support, in the spirit of Purusha's loving view of Prakriti. In our work with clients, we and/or our clients may find that emotions are stirred. We can give our clients the gift of witnessing this process, while they evolve through transformation—without trying to rush them or judge them. As we provide healing presence for the client, we are able to create the space for co-creation.

CONCLUSION

In this chapter, we reviewed why we are taking an evidence-informed approach to the co-creation of Yoga for One programs. We explored how the evidence-informed practice model is broader than an evidence-based one, as it links together the 3 Es: the client's lived *e*xperience, the *e*vidence base (both formative and empirical), and the *e*xpertise (of our field and of ourselves). We considered ways that a one-on-one yoga program can be approached from both the healthcare and public health points of view. Then, we explored a variety of ways we can conceptualize and enact the co-creation of a one-on-one yoga program, including the COACH framework for engaging with clients.

Let's turn next to how we can set up a healthy foundation for this program co-creation process, through the establishment of a solid business model. After that, we'll explore how we can attract our ideal client through the 9 Ps of marketing (Chapter 4); how we can meet the client where they are throughout the intake, interview, and assessment process (Chapter 5); and how we can co-create yoga programs and practices (Chapters 6 and 7). As you'll see, our inclusive and evidence-informed approach to co-creation is embedded throughout this entire journey!

CHAPTER 3

Building Your Program Foundation with a Business Model

When you co-create a one-on-one yoga program with your clients, you are providing them with a service within your scope of practice. Whether you do so through your own business or through another business as an independent contractor or employee, it is important to understand how the business model you are operating in enables this work to happen and impacts how it happens. In this chapter, we'll explore business models and consider how they can impact the co-creation of any one-on-one yoga program.

WHAT IS "BUSINESS VALUE?"

Most yoga professionals I have been honored to meet don't like thinking of their work as a business, because for them their work is about much more than money and profit. However, as noted by Eric Jorgenson (2015),[13] business is about generating value. Although many people think that businesses are profit-driven, many are, in actuality, purpose-driven. In this way, a business is an entity or endeavor that creates, delivers, and captures value for and from its stakeholders through its activities. This value can manifest in various forms:

- *Economic:* Often the most recognized form of value, economic value refers to monetary benefits. This includes profits for businesses, wages for employees, and products or services for customers at a price they find acceptable.

- *Social:* Businesses can contribute to society by creating jobs, fostering community development, engaging in corporate social responsibility (CSR) initiatives that address specific social issues, or promoting health and well-being.

- *Environmental:* In today's context of sustainability, businesses are increasingly seen as entities that can generate value by adopting eco-friendly practices, conserving resources, or producing goods and services that have a positive environmental impact.

- *Innovative:* Businesses drive innovation, introducing new products, services, or processes that can change markets or even everyday life. This kind of value can lead to improved efficiencies, better user experiences, or entirely new solutions to problems.

- *Cultural:* Some businesses contribute to cultural preservation, promotion, or evolution. This could be through the media they produce, the traditions they keep alive, or the new cultural norms they help shape.

- *Educational:* Businesses can offer educational resources, training, or experiences, equipping individuals with knowledge and skills that can be used in various facets of life.

- *Emotional:* Brands often aim to connect with their customers on an emotional level. This emotional bond can lead to brand loyalty, a sense of belonging, or a particular lifestyle that the customer values.

- *Operational:* For Business-to-Business (B2B) or for those in the supply chain, generating value can mean offering solutions that improve operational efficiency, reduce costs, or enhance the quality of processes for other businesses.

A solid business foundation equips a yoga program with the tools, resources, and stability to offer these teachings to the broadest possible audience, ensuring longevity, growth, and a lasting positive impact on its community.

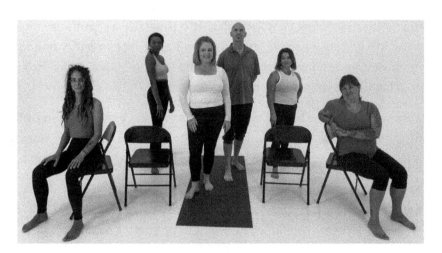

WHAT IS A "BUSINESS MODEL"?

A business model is a comprehensive framework that outlines how a business creates value, generates revenue, and operates to serve clients in a sustainable way. It serves as a blueprint for how a business conducts its operations, interacts with customers, and achieves its financial goals (see Figure 3).

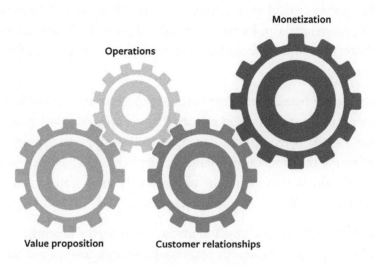

FIGURE 3: YOGA FOR ONE BUSINESS MODEL

UNDERSTANDING WHY BUSINESS MODELS MATTER FOR YOGA FOR ONE PROGRAMS

Operating a program with a strong business model foundation provides a more systematic, sustainable, and efficient approach compared to running it without a structured business framework. Here are several reasons why a strong business model foundation is important for businesses offering one-on-one yoga programs:

- *Clarity of purpose:* A solid business model provides clear direction and objectives. It establishes the program's value proposition, target market, and how it intends to reach and serve that market. A yoga professional who specializes in serving a particular niche can then clearly communicate this in marketing materials, ensuring the ideal clientele is reached, and that their specific needs are addressed.

- *Sustainability:* A business model outlines how a program will generate revenue, manage costs, and ultimately sustain itself over the long term. Without a business model, a program might not be able to ensure its ongoing viability. A one-on-one yoga instructor who has a set pricing strategy for classes, packages, and potential workshops can forecast income. For example, offering a discount for booking multiple sessions in advance could ensure a steady flow of revenue.

- *Resource allocation:* With a structured business approach, it's easier to determine where resources (time, money, workforce) should be allocated. This ensures that critical areas receive adequate attention and investment. A yoga professional can invest in specialized props for individual clients, or dedicate time to continuous learning, ensuring they're equipped to offer the best service.

- *Measurability and accountability:* Business models often come with key performance indicators (KPIs) and metrics to track progress. This allows for continuous assessment and ensures accountability in delivering promised value. Monitoring the progress of clients, perhaps through feedback or physical/mental health improvements, helps validate the effectiveness of the sessions and allows for adjustments where necessary.

- *Scalability:* A strong business foundation provides the blueprint for growth. It allows a program to identify opportunities for expansion, and provides the tools and strategies to scale effectively. For a business offering Yoga for One programs, scalability is possible through the growth of the practice (offering one-on-one yoga) and eventually through larger promotional and training efforts (such as online training courses, group sessions, or weekend retreats).

- *Risk management:* Operating within a business framework often involves identifying potential risks and devising strategies to mitigate them. This proactive approach can prevent or minimize challenges and disruptions. For example, insurance for potential injuries, contingency plans for no-show clients, and/or backup plans for outdoor sessions in case of bad weather can help mitigate business risks.

- *Client and partner confidence:* Partners often have greater confidence in a program that operates on a solid business foundation. It signals professionalism, foresight, and a commitment to long-term success. For one-on-one yoga providers, this makes a difference in terms of referrals from partners and clients. By showcasing testimonials and success stories, potential clients or partners, such as wellness centers, might be more willing to collaborate or refer clients.

- *Competitive advantage:* In a crowded market, having a well-thought-out business model can differentiate a program from its competitors, providing it with a unique value proposition or operational efficiency that sets it apart. Offering specialized techniques, like a unique meditation method or combining yoga with another modality (within the yoga professional's scope of practice), can set the yoga professional apart from competitors in the eyes of their ideal clients.

- *Legal and regulatory compliance:* Operating within a business framework often necessitates staying updated with relevant laws, regulations, and industry standards, ensuring the program remains compliant and avoids potential legal pitfalls. Ensuring certifications are up to date, obtaining necessary business licenses, and staying informed about health and safety regulations ensures the instructor operates legally and builds trust with clients.

As you can see, a strong business model foundation provides the necessary structure, strategy, and systems to maximize the program's potential. The business model provides the foundation for ensuring the longevity, growth, and positive impact of the business, so that the yoga professional has a stable base to serve value to clients.

VALUE PROPOSITION (WHY WE MAKE OUR CLIENTS' LIVES BETTER)

A value proposition is a short-and-sweet statement that communicates how a business will solve client problems and deliver value. Written in a clear and concise way that is easy to understand, it explains what the overall aims are for a business from a client-centered point of view. A well-crafted value proposition is focused on the ideal client's needs, problems, and desires; it explains how the business can help the client to solve their perceived problems through the use of the business's products and/or services.

From a socio-ecological perspective (see Chapter 2), a Yoga for One program generates value at the individual, interpersonal, interprofessional, and societal (population health) level:

- *At the individual level,* a Yoga for One program's value proposition is found in the unique way that each program supports each client in solving their current problems and achieving their unique vision and goals through the unique perspective and scope of practice of the yoga professional co-creating the program.

- *At the interpersonal level*, a Yoga for One program's value proposition is found in the co-creation process of shared decision-making and the social support that clients receive through support from their Yoga for One provider.

- *At the interprofessional level*, a Yoga for One program's value proposition is based on the yoga professional's scope of practice. For example, a yoga coach offers the value proposition of behavior change, motivation, and accountability support. A yoga teacher offers the value proposition of health and yoga education, improved yoga literacy, and goal-centered work focused on the client's health and fitness goals. A yoga therapist offers the value proposition of a yoga program that is individualized for the client's medical needs and concerns and aligned for their health and well-being goals.

- *At the societal (population health) level*, a Yoga for One program's value proposition is found in the ripple effect created by each program's delivery. As discussed in Chapter 2, the individual's results can spark a ripple effect out to the other socio-ecological levels, thereby making an impact on overall population health.

As we can see, the articulation of the value proposition changes based on which stakeholder group (socio-ecological level) we are focused on. In this way, a value proposition can play a crucial role in Yoga for One promotional efforts, such as advertising, websites, marketing materials, and sales pitches, to attract new customers.

Let's co-create your value proposition

A value proposition clarifies why someone should choose your yoga services over another, and encapsulates the unique benefits and features of the service provided. A strong value proposition is clear, specific, and speaks directly to the needs and desires of your ideal clients in a compelling way.

SELF-REFLECTION: YOUR UNIQUE QUALITIES

Credentials and training:

- List your certifications, training programs, and any special courses you've completed.
- Are you specialized in any specific type of yoga (e.g., hatha, vinyasa, prenatal)?

Experience:

- How many years have you been practicing yoga?
- How many years have you been teaching yoga?

Personal strengths:

- List 3–5 personal strengths that enhance your teaching (e.g., patience, adaptability, deep anatomical knowledge).

Outline your ideal client's needs and pain points
Ideal client:

- Who are you aiming to serve (e.g., beginners, athletes, seniors, people recovering from injuries)?

Pain points:

- List common problems or challenges faced by your target audience.
- How does yoga address these pain points?

Itemize your offerings and solutions
Service differentiators:

- What makes your training sessions unique compared to other yoga trainers?
- Do you offer something that most don't (e.g., personalized sequences, flexible timing, holistic wellness advice)?

Compare your offerings with the competition

- Identify 2–3 other yoga professionals in your area.
- Review their value propositions and business models.
- How could you differentiate yourself from them?

Summarize your value proposition

Using the information gathered above, draft a concise value proposition statement. For example:

> I am a certified hatha yoga teacher with five years of experience in working with clients one-on-one to help them to get back their mobility after injury. I specialize in helping people who want to have a yoga program tailored to their unique and individual health needs, so they can return to mobility safely while experiencing peace of mind.

Value proposition tips

- Revisit and revise your value proposition as you gain more experience, gather more feedback, or shift your focus. Keep it concise, and focus on the most compelling points.

- Use your value proposition in marketing materials, on your website, and when discussing your services with potential clients.

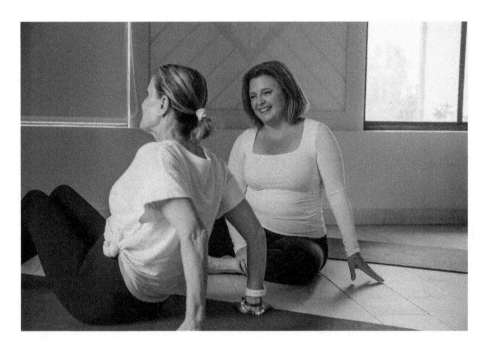

MONETIZATION (HOW WE GENERATE REVENUE)

While the value proposition is the strategy through which a business generates value with its customer/s, monetization is the strategy through which a business generates revenue (profit). Interestingly, this is true for both non-profit and for-profit businesses. In the case of a non-profit business, or not-for-profit business, generated revenue is invested back into the business to support its mission. In the case of a for-profit business, generated revenue is distributed to the owner/s of the business. As you can see, monetization matters for any type of business.

Understanding monetization

At its core, monetization pertains to the strategies or methods a company employs to generate profit from its assets. This term embodies the overarching approach detailing how a business can transform its various offerings into tangible cash.

Like yoga, monetization is holistic, and inclusive of all assets, from intellectual property to tangible goods, and finding diverse ways to derive income from them. For instance, a tech company can monetize its proprietary software through licensing agreements; a blogger can monetize their platform through affiliate marketing; and a yoga professional can monetize their capacity to provide one-on-one yoga programs by promoting them directly to clients or by securing a third party grant to fund these programs with underserved populations. For yoga professionals, monetization is the bridge between passionate teaching and financial stability.

The essence of monetization is to determine how value can be translated into profit. In the case of a Yoga for One program, this could mean determining the cost of the program, introducing multiple payment options, effectively communicating with clients to convert potential leads into paying ones, and keeping track of metrics of success.

Several tactical activities fall under the umbrella of a monetization strategy:

- *Pricing strategy*: Setting the right price is vital. The strategy can involve tiered pricing, freemium models, dynamic pricing, subscription models, or one-time fees. The pricing should reflect the value provided, market demand, and competitive landscape.

- *Payment infrastructure*: Having a secure, user-friendly payment system in place is necessary to collect revenue. This includes payment gateways, e-commerce platforms, and subscription management tools.

- *Distribution channels:* These are the avenues through which products or services are sold. It could be direct sales via a company website, through app stores, affiliate marketing, third party retailers, or physical stores.

- *Sales and marketing strategies:* Effective promotion and sales tactics are crucial to drive awareness and convince potential customers of the value being offered.

- *Protection of intellectual property:* Especially important for digital goods, patents, copyrights, trademarks, and trade secrets can protect a company's unique offerings, allowing them to monetize without immediate threats from imitators.

- *Customer engagement and retention:* The initial sale is just the beginning. Strategies to keep customers engaged, like loyalty programs or continuous content updates, can lead to longer-term monetization through repeat purchases or subscriptions.

- *Feedback and analytics:* Tracking and analyzing customer behavior, sales data, and feedback helps in refining the monetization strategies, allowing businesses to adapt and maximize revenue.

- *Regulatory and compliance considerations:* Ensuring all monetization efforts adhere to local and international laws, including taxation, data privacy, and consumer rights, is essential to avoid penalties and maintain a positive brand reputation.

- *Scalability:* The monetization strategy should be scalable. As the business grows, the methods of generating revenue should be able to expand and evolve without major overhauls.

- *Diversification:* Relying on a single revenue stream can be risky. Successful monetization often involves diversifying how a business earns, tapping into multiple revenue streams to ensure stability.

As we can see, monetization is not just about making money! These components, when effectively combined, can lead to a robust monetization strategy that maximizes revenue while delivering value to the customer.

Payment models (income)

In the operation of a yoga or health business, it is important to recognize that there are unique payment models that can be applied to the funding of a Yoga for One program. These payment models—also referred to as revenue streams—bring income to the business. Let's explore the most common payment models that are possible for a Yoga for One program.

Fee-for-service (FFS) model

The FFS model is the one most frequently used in the professional delivery of yoga. In this model, those receiving care (clients) pay the person or organization delivering the service directly for each service they receive. This model may not promote cost-effective care for the client, because the services are not subsidized. In everyday language, this is the "out of pocket" model because clients are paying themselves for the care they receive without reimbursement. The FFS model covers the following:

- *One-time payment:* This is a straightforward model where a customer pays a single, upfront fee for a product or service. Examples include buying a physical product in a store or paying for a software license. In the case of a Yoga for One program, this model would be used when a client pays for their initial consultation visit for a program package.

- *Subscription model:* Customers pay a recurring fee at regular intervals (e.g., monthly, annually) to access a product or service. This model is common for services like streaming platforms (e.g., Netflix, Spotify) or SaaS (Software as a Service) applications. In the case of a Yoga for One program, this model could be used with a client who wants to receive ongoing and regular program delivery and access, or when they pay for a month-to-month service (such as a membership).

- *Pay-per-use/consumption:* Customers are charged based on their actual usage or consumption of a product or service. In the case of a Yoga for One program, this model could be used with a client who wants to be charged based on actual attendance at sessions, rather than a monthly or annually based program.

- *Freemium model:* This model combines free and premium offerings. Basic features or services are offered for free to attract users, while premium features or services are available for a fee. Companies often use this model in mobile apps and online games. In the case of a Yoga for One program, this model could be used when a yoga professional offers initial content and/or value in an asynchronous way (such as YouTube or an app), and then invites the client to continue with additional features of the program for a fee.

- *Tiered pricing:* In this model, customers can choose from different tiers or levels of a product or service, each offering a different set of features or capabilities at varying price points. This is common in software and online services. In the case of a Yoga for One program, this is used to generate a value ladder of offerings with increasing levels of live one-on-one support. (We will discuss this model further in Chapter 4.)

- *Bundled payments:* In a bundled payment model, a single payment is made for a group of related services or procedures that are typically delivered during an episode of care. This approach encourages coordination among different providers, and can lead to cost savings and improved quality of care. In the case of a Yoga for One program, a client may invest in a training series with a studio and receive access to classes as well as their Yoga for One program.

- *Direct primary care (DPC):* In a DPC model, patients pay a monthly or annual fee to a primary care provider for a defined set of services. This eliminates the need for FFS billing, and can lead to longer, more comprehensive visits with primary care providers. In a Yoga for One program, this model could be applied by offering an annual access fee for program co-creation services and support.

- *Episode-of-care payments:* This model involves making a single payment for all services related to a specific medical condition or episode of care, from diagnosis to recovery. It encourages cost-effective and coordinated care. In a Yoga for One program, this would work well in an allied healthcare or wellness setting, in which the yoga program would be combined with other services in support of the client's comprehensive care plan.

Performance-based models

Traditionally, healthcare providers were reimbursed based on the number of services they rendered, irrespective of the results. However, with rising healthcare costs and the necessity for improved patient outcomes, newer models of payment have emerged. Two pivotal approaches in this paradigm shift are the pay-for-performance (P4P) or quality measurement and value-based purchasing (VBP) models. Both strive to link provider compensation more closely to the quality of care delivered, ensuring that patients receive the best possible outcomes at a justifiable cost:

- *Pay-for-performance (P4P) or quality measurement:* P4P models tie a portion of provider payments to specific quality and outcome measures. Providers earn additional payments if they meet or exceed performance targets related to patient outcomes, patient satisfaction, or other quality metrics.

- *Value-based purchasing* (VBP): This combines elements of P4P and quality measurement. Providers are rewarded or penalized based on the value of care they deliver, considering both cost and quality. This model aims to align payment with the overall value of care provided.

Population-based models

Some payment models aim to strike a balance between offering top-notch care and maintaining fiscal responsibility. These models aim to enhance patient outcomes while also controlling expenditure by introducing unique mechanisms to align provider incentives with patient-centered, value-driven care. The following are the three most common population-based models:

- *Capitation:* Under capitation, healthcare providers are paid a fixed amount per patient per month (or year) regardless of the services provided. This model encourages providers to focus on preventive care and cost-effective treatments because they have a financial incentive to keep their patients healthy.

- *Shared savings and accountable care organizations (ACOs):* ACOs are groups of healthcare providers that work together to coordinate care for a defined patient population. They may share in the savings achieved by providing high-quality, cost-effective care. This model promotes care coordination and population health management.

- *Global payment:* Also known as population-based or global budget payment, this model assigns a fixed budget to a healthcare organization to cover all the healthcare needs of a defined population. The organization is responsible for managing costs and improving health outcomes within that budget.

Cost structure (expenses)

As we have learned, monetization is focused on the generation of revenue. It is important to remember that revenue is not generated by income; it is generated through profit. This means that it is important to consider what costs (expenses) are also required to operate a yoga business. These costs can be categorized into fixed and variable costs:

Examples of fixed costs:

- Rent or facility costs

- Compensation (salaries and contractor fees)

- Insurance

- Utilities and maintenance

- Equipment and props

- Software and technology

- Professional development

- Business licenses and permits

- Legal and accounting services.

Examples of variable costs:

- Session materials

- Marketing and promotion

- Client acquisition

- Travel expenses

- Client amenities

- Payment processing fees.

Cost of goods sold (COGS)

COGS refers to the direct costs associated with producing or delivering the goods (in this case, services) offered by a business. In the context of a one-on-one yoga business, where the primary service is providing personalized yoga instruction, the COGS may not be as significant as in a product-based business. Examples of COGS include:

- Yoga props and equipment

- Session materials

- Client amenities

- Health and safety supplies.

Understanding net profit

As its name implies, net profit is a clear indicator of a business's profitability (revenue generated). Understanding monetization from a net profit perspective is crucial for sustainable business operations and growth; it's not just about earning more, but also about efficiently managing expenses to maximize the profit margin. By strategically diversifying revenue streams, optimizing costs, and regularly reviewing the financial health of the business, a Yoga for One professional can aim to ensure their passion aligns with profitability. Options include:

- *Diversify revenue streams:* Instead of relying solely on one-on-one sessions, group classes, online sessions, or workshops can be offered. By having multiple revenue streams, the impact of a decline in one particular area can be mitigated.

- *Optimize pricing:* Regularly evaluate and adjust pricing based on market demand, expertise level, and client feedback. An occasional rate increase, especially as you gain more experience or training, can significantly boost revenue.

- *Minimize overheads:* Efficiently managing fixed costs like studio rent or utility bills can have a direct positive impact on net profit. Consider sharing studio space, moving to a more cost-effective location, or even offering outdoor sessions.

- *Utilize digital platforms:* Offering online classes, webinars, or on-demand video content can cater to a broader audience with minimal incremental costs, enhancing the net profit margin.

- *Sell merchandise:* Selling yoga-related products, such as mats, apparel, or even branded accessories, can serve as an additional revenue source. Ensure the markup on these products accounts for all associated costs to ensure profitability.

- *Efficient marketing:* Instead of broad-spectrum advertising, focus on targeted marketing efforts. Utilize social media, engage in local community events, or employ word-of-mouth referrals, which might offer a higher return on investment than traditional advertising.

- *Regularly review expenses:* Periodically analyze all business expenses to identify any redundant or excessive costs. This could include renegotiating contracts or finding alternative suppliers for necessary services or products.

- *Tax efficiency:* Understand local tax regulations and take advantage of any permissible deductions, rebates, or incentives. Working with a financial advisor or accountant can ensure you're not overpaying on taxes.

- *Offer packages or memberships:* Instead of single-session pricing, offer package deals or memberships. This not only ensures consistent revenue, but also builds client loyalty.

For a yoga professional, monetization can be challenging, but it is achievable. Understanding and adeptly maneuvering through these aspects can ensure a sustainable and profitable career.

CUSTOMER RELATIONSHIPS (WHO WE SERVE)

Customer relationships, particularly in the context of a one-on-one yoga professional, play a pivotal role in shaping the overall business model. The depth, quality, and nature of the relationship between the yoga professional and their client can significantly influence success. Here's an explanation of why customer relationships are a key component of a business model for a one-on-one yoga professional:

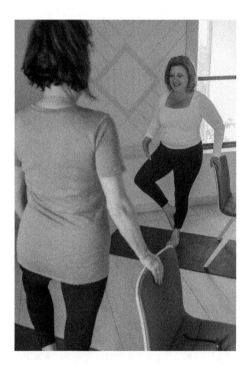

- *Trust and rapport:* One-on-one yoga sessions are private experiences where clients often share personal health information, physical limitations, and personal goals. A strong customer relationship built on trust ensures that clients feel safe, understood, and comfortable enough to be themselves and to share their story during sessions.

- *Personalization:* Understanding each client's unique needs, preferences, and progress allows the yoga professional to tailor sessions, ensuring they are effective and meaningful. This level of personalization can only be achieved through a deep understanding cultivated through a strong customer relationship.

- *Client retention:* Consistent and positive interactions foster loyalty. When clients feel valued and notice tangible benefits from their sessions, they are more likely to continue their lessons, ensuring a steady revenue stream for the professional.

- *Word-of-mouth referrals:* Satisfied clients often share their positive experiences with friends, family, and colleagues. Strong customer relationships can thus lead to organic growth through referrals, minimizing marketing costs, and attracting clients who are already inclined to trust the yoga professional based on personal recommendations.

- *Feedback and improvement:* A close relationship with clients encourages open dialogue. Clients are more likely to provide honest feedback, allowing the yoga professional to make necessary adjustments to their teaching methods, techniques, or even business operations.

- *Pricing flexibility:* Trusting relationships can allow for more flexible pricing strategies, such as package deals or loyalty discounts. Clients who perceive high value and have a strong relationship with their yoga professional might be willing to invest more in long-term packages or premium services.

- *Emotional support:* Beyond the physical practice, yoga often delves into emotional and mental well-being. A strong customer relationship allows the yoga professional to offer emotional support, deepening the holistic benefits of the sessions.

- *Crisis management:* In any business, unforeseen challenges may arise—scheduling conflicts, misunderstandings, or even potential grievances. A robust customer relationship can facilitate smoother negotiations and resolutions during such times.

- *Community building:* Strong individual relationships can lay the foundation for building a broader community. This can lead to group sessions, workshops, or retreats, expanding the yoga professional's offerings and reach.

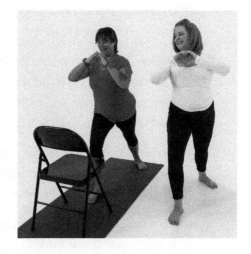

For a one-on-one yoga professional, the essence of the business goes beyond just the physical practice; it's deeply rooted in the interpersonal dynamics between the yoga professional and the client. Cultivating and nurturing these customer relationships not only enhances the immediate yoga experience, but also drives the long-term viability and growth of the professional's business.

Key partnerships

In a yoga business model, customer relationships do not only occur with clients and students. Key partnerships can play a crucial role in supporting the business foundation needed to deliver one-on-one yoga programs, by expanding reach, enhancing credibility, and offering additional support and resources. Here are some key partnerships that may serve to strengthen a business model, by supporting you, the yoga professional, in your relationship with your clients:

- *Yoga studios and wellness centers:* Collaborate with local yoga studios and wellness centers to offer one-on-one sessions to clients. Partnering with established studios can help in accessing a broader audience and leverage an existing client base.

- *Medical practitioners and healthcare providers:* Establish partnerships with healthcare professionals, such as physicians, physical therapists, chiropractors, and mental health therapists. These healthcare professionals can refer clients to your yoga therapy program as a complementary or alternative therapy for specific health conditions.

- *Holistic health practitioners:* Partner with practitioners in complementary fields, such as nutritionists, herbalists, massage therapists, and acupuncturists. Together, you can offer holistic wellness packages that address clients' physical, mental, and emotional well-being.

- *Corporate wellness programs:* Collaborate with companies and organizations to provide one-on-one yoga sessions as part of their employee wellness programs. Workplace wellness partnerships can offer a steady stream of clients.

- *Fitness and sports centers:* Partner with fitness centers, sports clubs, or athletic organizations to offer yoga for athletes, injury prevention, or recovery programs. Athletes and active individuals can benefit from personalized yoga instruction.

- *Online platforms and marketplaces:* List your one-on-one yoga or yoga therapy services on online marketplaces and wellness directories. These platforms can help you reach a broader online audience.

- *Yoga teacher training schools:* Collaborate with yoga teacher training programs to offer specialized workshops or certifications in yoga therapy. This partnership can help you train future yoga therapists and instructors.

- *Educational institutions:* Partner with schools, colleges, or universities to offer yoga therapy programs for students, faculty, or staff. Yoga can support stress management and overall well-being among academic communities.

- *Community and support groups:* Collaborate with local community organizations, support groups, or recovery centers. Offer one-on-one yoga or yoga therapy sessions tailored to the specific needs of these groups, such as trauma survivors or individuals dealing with addiction.

- *Online influencers and wellness bloggers:* Partner with influencers and wellness bloggers in the digital space who can promote your services to their followers. Influencers can provide testimonials and reviews, increasing your program's visibility.

- *Professional associations:* Join and become active in professional associations related to yoga, therapy, and wellness. Networking within these organizations can lead to valuable partnerships and referrals.

- *Local businesses:* Establish partnerships with local businesses, such as spas, beauty salons, or health food stores. Offer discounts or joint promotions to attract clients from these establishments.

- *Non-profit organizations:* Collaborate with non-profit organizations focused on health and well-being. Offer your services for community events, workshops, or fundraising activities.

- *Media outlets:* Partner with local media outlets, including newspapers, magazines, and radio stations, for interviews, articles, or advertising opportunities. Media exposure can help raise awareness of your programs.

- *Professional therapists and counselors:* Partner with mental health therapists, counselors, or psychologists. Yoga therapy can complement their treatment plans for clients dealing with stress, anxiety, or trauma.

Effective partnerships require clear communication, shared goals, and mutual benefits. When forming these relationships, it's essential to align your offerings with the needs and objectives of your partners to create win-win situations that promote your one-on-one yoga and yoga therapy programs.

OPERATIONS (WHAT WE DO TO SERVE OUR CUSTOMERS)

If the value proposition is the "why" of the business, monetization is the "how" of the business, and customer relationships is the "who" of the business, then operations is the "what" of the business. A yoga personal trainer business, like any other enterprise, requires a well-structured operational framework to thrive. Operating beyond the realm of group classes, a personal yoga trainer offers specialized, one-on-one sessions tailored to individual needs.

Efficient and streamlined operations ensure that the value proposition is reliably delivered, monetization strategies are effectively executed, and customer relationships are consistently nurtured. To ensure the efficiency and sustainability of such a venture, understanding and addressing its operational needs is paramount. Here is an in-depth exploration of these needs:

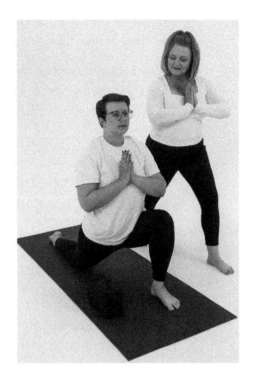

- *Client management system:* Efficiently managing client details, their health backgrounds, specific goals, and progress over time is essential. A robust client management system or software can streamline this, ensuring that client details are readily accessible, schedules don't overlap, and progress is tracked systematically.

- *Scheduling and booking:* Given that personal training often works on appointments, an efficient booking system is crucial. This could be a digital solution allowing clients to see availability and book sessions, or a manual approach where the yoga professional manages the calendar. Regardless, it should avoid double bookings, consider buffer time between sessions, and send reminders to clients.

- *Space and equipment:* A serene, clean, and well-equipped space is vital. Depending on the clientele, this could be a home studio, a rented space, or even a mobile solution where the yoga professional visits the client's chosen location. The environment should be conducive to yoga, possibly with essential props like yoga mats, blocks, straps, and bolsters.

- *Financial management:* From setting pricing structures to managing expenses and ensuring timely payments, financial operations are the backbone of sustainability. This includes invoicing, tracking payments, managing business expenses, and accounting for taxes.

- *Marketing and outreach*: Operations aren't just about managing the existing client base but also about reaching potential clients. This involves marketing strategies, managing an online presence through a website or social media, and engaging in community outreach or partnerships.

- *Continuous learning and certification*: The world of yoga is vast and ever evolving. Yoga professionals must invest in ongoing education, attend workshops, and possibly acquire advanced certifications. This ensures that they offer the latest and most beneficial techniques to their clients.

- *Feedback and improvement*: Operational efficiency requires continuous feedback. Regularly soliciting client feedback can help identify areas of improvement, adjust techniques, or introduce new offerings.

- *Health and safety protocols*: Ensuring the physical well-being of clients is paramount. This includes understanding any medical concerns or injuries a client might have, ensuring safe practices, and possibly having liability insurance. In today's context, hygiene and cleanliness, especially in shared spaces, have also become significant operational concerns.

- *Digital integration*: In the era of technology, many yoga professionals have expanded their offerings to online sessions, especially given global situations like the Covid-19 pandemic. This requires operational adjustments such as reliable internet connectivity, video conferencing tools, and potentially, digital payment solutions.

- *Legal compliance*: Depending on the region, there might be specific legal requirements for operating a personal training business. This could involve business registration, obtaining necessary permits, and ensuring that all services offered comply with local regulations.

- *Personal well-being*: Lastly, but most importantly, yoga professionals need to ensure their well-being. This includes managing their schedules to prevent burnout, investing in self-care, and maintaining their yoga practice. After all, a trainer's personal energy and health directly influence the quality of training provided.

By understanding and efficiently managing these operational needs, a yoga personal trainer can not only offer exceptional service to their clients, but also ensure the longevity and success of their business.

CONCLUSION

As you can see, a business model isn't just a static plan on paper; it's a dynamic and holistic representation of how a company functions and thrives in the competitive marketplace. By cohesively integrating the value proposition, monetization strategies, and daily operations, a company can ensure its longevity, profitability, and relevance in its industry. This integrated approach not only captures the essence of what a business stands for, but also delineates the path it charts for future growth and success.

CHAPTER 4

Social Marketing

AN INCLUSIVE APPROACH TO YOUR MARKETING MIX

Many yoga professionals find themselves in the same conundrum I faced for many years. On the one hand, I didn't like the idea that I had to sell my work, and I felt like I was "selling out" when I did. On the other hand, I wanted to share yoga with as many people as I could and knew that they needed to "buy in" to what it could offer them. Eventually, this conundrum led me to pursue a PhD in health communication, so that I could study health promotion as a science. Over time, I explored various ways I could ease the dis-ease I had within myself—the lack of ease I had in regard to promoting yoga.

In this chapter, I will share my approach to promoting yoga—which has taken 10 years to develop. As you'll see, it is grounded in a social marketing approach. Ultimately, I hope that this approach helps you, too, to ease the dis-ease that can come with the promotion of a one-on-one program, so that you can promote your client's buy-in without the same sense of dis-ease I had for so many years.

WHY A SOCIAL MARKETING APPROACH MAKES SENSE FOR YOGA PROFESSIONALS

Social marketing utilizes marketing principles to foster behaviors or attitudes that benefit both society and the individual: "Social marketing is an approach used to develop activities aimed at changing or maintaining people's behavior for the benefit of individuals and society as a whole."[14]

Through the application of commercial marketing principles and techniques, social marketing aims to bring about positive societal change and influence behavior. In the same way that marketing campaigns spotlight our "pain points" and then convince consumers that their product or service can alleviate the problem, social marketing campaigns highlight societal or individual challenges and offer a mindset, behavior, or societal change as the remedy.

A social marketing approach aligns well with our goal of inclusivity in promoting a one-on-one yoga program. Through a social marketing strategy, we can stay consumer-focused in keeping with the central tenets (principles) of person-centered care. We can create compelling invitations for the client to let go of competing demands so that they can engage in our program—and ultimately achieve their personal health and well-being goals. We can encourage prospective clients to progress through a behavior change process that supports their program engagement journey rather than pushing them too fast into program adoption. We can build trust over time as part of our overarching efforts to make yoga more accessible and attainable for all.

Marketing efforts aim to transform prospectors into evangelists and strangers into stakeholders—who not only love working with you, but are also the first to recommend you and your program. In this section we will explore how you can think about, plan for, and implement your social marketing approach in a cohesive way—otherwise known as a marketing mix.

MEET MY MARKETING 9 PS

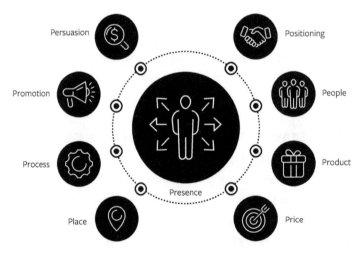

FIGURE 4: YOGA FOR ONE 9 PS OF THE MARKETING MIX

Today, when you say "marketing mix" to marketing and business professionals, they will know exactly what you are referring to: *product, price, place (distribution)*, and *promotion*, or, as they are more commonly called, the *4 Ps*.

Based on my experience promoting, co-creating, and delivering programs, I have expanded these 4 Ps into what I call the 9 Ps of the social marketing mix for one-on-one yoga programs. These are the nine elements we can consider in marketing one-on-one yoga programs: *presence, positioning, people, product, price, place (distribution), process (improvement), promotion,* and *persuasion* (see Figure 4). Let's explore what I mean by each of these, and how you can apply them in the development of your own marketing mix, for the marketing of any product and/or service, including your Yoga for One programs.

P1 Presence: holding space for healing

Healing presence has been described as an "interpersonal, intrapersonal, and transpersonal to transcendent phenomenon that leads to a beneficial, therapeutic, and/or positive spiritual change within another individual (healee) and also within the healer."[15]

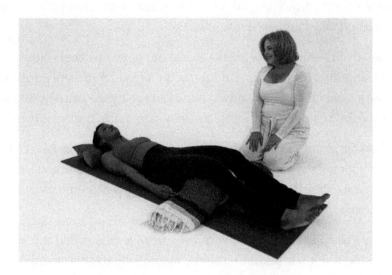

In the co-creation of a one-on-one yoga program, healing presence refers to the deep, holistic, and oftentimes spiritual connections we establish as yoga professionals with our clients. It goes beyond mere physical presence and encompasses emotional, psychological, and sometimes spiritual attunement to the individual. Through healing presence, we can enact our one-on-one yoga program intention of inclusivity, because when individuals feel safe and trust their caregivers, they are more likely to engage actively in their care, communicate openly about their needs, and adhere to therapeutic recommendations.[16]

It is my belief that healing presence does not begin when we meet the client and begin delivering their Yoga for One program. Instead, I believe healing presence begins when we begin engaging with prospective clients through our marketing efforts. If we stay grounded in the space of healing presence when we promote ourselves, our clients' first impression of us will be grounded in this presence too. In this way, we are beginning to co-create the healing presence dynamic before we have even met the client.

Here are a few ways that intentionality towards healing presence can benefit our marketing efforts:

- *Deepens client connection:* In a market saturated with yoga instructors and classes, healing presence can set an instructor apart. Clients tend to gravitate towards teachers who make them feel seen, heard, and understood. Such connections often lead to long-term student–teacher relationships.

- *Enhances word-of-mouth recommendations:* Clients who experience genuine care and attention are more likely to share their positive experiences with friends and family. Personal recommendations can be a potent marketing tool, especially in the wellness industry.

- *Builds trust:* For many, yoga is not just about physical fitness but also mental and emotional well-being. An instructor's healing presence fosters trust, ensuring clients feel safe and supported in their yoga journey, which can be crucial for newcomers or for those using yoga for therapeutic reasons.

- *Allows for personalized adjustments:* A strong sense of presence enables the instructor to intuitively adjust sessions based on a client's mood, energy levels, and needs on any given day. This tailored approach enhances the overall experience and perceived value.

- *Boosts retention rates:* When clients feel a genuine connection and see tangible benefits from their sessions, they're more likely to continue their journey with the same instructor, leading to consistent revenue.

- *Enhances brand reputation:* A yoga instructor or studio known for its healing presence can become synonymous with holistic well-being, setting a gold standard in the industry.

- *Supports authentic marketing:* In an age where consumers are wary of overly polished or scripted marketing messages, genuine testimonials and narratives about an instructor's healing presence can resonate more deeply, drawing in like-minded clients.

- *Facilitates emotional healing:* For many individuals, yoga is a tool for emotional healing. An instructor's healing presence can create a safe space for clients to release emotional blockages, enhancing the transformative power of the sessions.

- *Elevates the overall experience:* Beyond just poses and techniques, the essence of yoga lies in the holistic experience. An instructor's healing presence elevates the entire practice, making it more profound and impactful.

- *Aligns with yoga's core philosophy:* At its heart, yoga is about union—of mind, body, and spirit. An instructor embodying a healing presence is living the true essence of yoga, making their offerings more authentic and aligned with the ancient practice's core philosophy.

Incorporating the concept of "healing presence" into marketing material can communicate the deeper value and transformative potential of the one-on-one yoga program, distinguishing it from more generic or commercialized offerings.

P2 Positioning: niche identification

The term "positioning" refers to the ways that a business or a program brands itself, and co-creates a distinct perception in the minds of potential and current clients. By effectively positioning themselves, one-on-one yoga teachers can attract clients who resonate with and value their unique offerings, thereby building a loyal client base.

A niche is a specialized segment of the market, catering to a specific group of people with particular interests, needs, or goals. In the context of a one-on-one yoga program, niche identification means honing in on a specific area, style, or group of individuals that you want to tailor your one-on-one program for. This niche could be based on a particular style of yoga, catering to a specific demographic (e.g., prenatal yoga, yoga for athletes), or even combining yoga with other holistic practices.

Why you should identify your niche

- *Stand out in the crowd:* The world of yoga is vast, with many yoga professionals offering a variety of styles and approaches. This can feel overwhelming to a new yoga practitioner, who doesn't yet understand all of the many options that they have to practice. By choosing a specific niche, you differentiate yourself within this large field of yoga, and make it easier for potential clients to find and choose you.

- *Deepen your expertise:* Specializing allows you to delve deeper into a particular area, enhancing your knowledge and skills. This focused expertise can make your sessions more impactful and valuable to your clients.

- *Tailored marketing and communication:* With a clear niche, your marketing efforts become more streamlined. You'll know exactly who your target audience is, what their needs are, and how to communicate with them effectively.

- *Higher client retention:* When clients feel that you offer something unique that caters specifically to their needs, they are more likely to stick with you long term.

- *Foster genuine connections:* By focusing on a niche, you attract clients who genuinely resonate with your approach. This alignment can lead to deeper, more meaningful connections during your sessions.

- *Optimized resource allocation:* Instead of spreading yourself thin trying to cater to everyone, you can invest your time, energy, and resources into perfecting your niche offering. This can lead to better results and higher satisfaction for both you and your clients.

Identifying a niche isn't about limiting yourself; it's about focusing your energy where it can have the most significant impact. For one-on-one yoga programs, where the connection between teacher and client is paramount, having a clear niche can enhance this bond, making each session more effective and fulfilling. Take some time to reflect on your passions and strengths, and the needs of the community around you. Finding your niche will not only elevate your practice but also enrich the lives of those you teach.

There are four ways we can approach niche identification: demographics, psychographics, practice readiness, and geography:

- *Demographic segmentation:* Dividing customers based on demographic factors like age, gender, income, education, and marital status, while maintaining our commitment to inclusivity:

  - *Age:* Creating segments based on age groups, such as teens, young adults, middle-aged individuals, and seniors.
  - *Gender:* Segmenting clients by gender identity, as some may prefer gender-specific classes while others may prefer gender-neutral classes. Honoring all gender identities is in keeping with our commitment to inclusivity.

    – *Income:* Offering different pricing options for programs based on income levels. Third party funding can offset pricing restraints, so that those who are unable to invest in the program based on income can receive a subsidy or full waiver.

- *Psychographic segmentation:* Segmenting based on psychological traits, values, interests, and lifestyles:

    – *Lifestyle and wellness goals:* Segmenting clients based on their values, beliefs, lifestyle choices, and overarching program aims. For example, some may be focused on more holistic wellness, while others may be focused on physical fitness.

    – *Interests:* Identifying clients with specific interests related to yoga, such as yoga for support for a particular hobby (e.g., yoga for golf or yoga for writers).

    – *Stress reduction:* Segmenting clients seeking stress relief, relaxation, or mindfulness practices.

    – *Fitness and weight management:* Tailoring programs for those interested in yoga as a fitness or weight management tool.

    – *Mental health and emotional well-being:* Addressing the needs of clients using yoga to improve mental health or emotional balance.

    – *Yoga style preferences:* Recognizing that clients may have preferences for specific yoga styles and offering classes accordingly, such as hatha, vinyasa, Ashtanga, yin, restorative, nidra, and meditation.

- *Practice readiness segmentation:* Segmenting based on the individual's yoga literacy (as described in Chapter 2) and practice readiness:

    – *Motivation:* Differentiating between clients who are primarily motivated by physical fitness, mental well-being, spiritual growth, or a combination of these.

    – *Experience and skill level:* Beginner, intermediate, and advanced, offering classes tailored to participants' experience levels, such as beginner-friendly or advanced yoga sessions.

    – *Specialty classes:* Segmenting by specialty needs, such as prenatal yoga, yoga for seniors, or therapeutic yoga for injury recovery.

    – *Scheduling and availability:* Morning, afternoon, and evening, offering classes at different times of the day to accommodate various schedules.

    – *Weekdays vs. weekends:* Catering to clients who prefer weekday or weekend yoga sessions.

- *Geographic segmentation:* Dividing customers based on geographic location, such as country, region, city, or climate:

  - *Online vs. in-person preferences:* Recognizing clients who prefer in-person classes and those who prefer online yoga sessions.
  - *Location-based classes:* Offering classes in specific locations or neighborhoods, especially in densely populated areas.

- *Special events and workshops:* Organizing special events, workshops, or retreats for dedicated segments, such as weekend yoga retreats for enthusiasts.

As you can see, there are many ways to identify and segment the niche you would like to serve with one-on-one yoga programs. One way to make this process meaningful and client-centered is to create an "ideal client avatar." This is essentially a personification of your market niche, embodied into a fictitious individual.

Although at first glance it may seem relatively easy to create a client avatar, the process can take time and deserves caution. In the process of creating an avatar, I recommend that you employ sensitivity and awareness to the DEIAB principles of diversity, equity, inclusion, access, and belonging (discussed in Chapter 2). We want to ensure that we aren't promoting stereotypes, being culturally insensitive, or making assumptions based on implicit bias.

Let's review several example ideal client avatars for one-on-one programs, detailing their demographics and psychographics as well as their challenges, goals, and preferences for yoga. These characteristics are then transformed into value propositions for each.

Avatar 1, Stress relief seeker Sarah[17]

- Demographics:

  - Age: 32
  - Gender: Female
  - Occupation: Corporate professional
  - Income: Middle to upper-middle class.

- Psychographics:

  - Experiences high stress and anxiety due to work and daily life
  - Seeking relaxation, mindfulness, and stress relief
  - Interested in improving mental and emotional well-being.

- Yoga preferences:

  - Prefers gentle and restorative yoga styles
  - Values meditation and breathing exercises
  - Flexible scheduling for early morning or evening sessions.

- Goals:

  - Reduce stress and anxiety
  - Improve sleep quality
  - Enhance overall mental and emotional well-being.

Avatar 2, Injury recovery Ian

- Demographics:

  - Age: 58
  - Gender: Male
  - Occupation: Semi-retired
  - Income: Varied.

- Psychographics:

  - Dealing with physical injuries caused by pickleball
  - Wants to regain mobility and reduce pain
  - May have limited previous experience with yoga.

- Yoga preferences:

  - Needs gentle, therapeutic, and rehabilitative yoga
  - Appreciates personalized attention and adjustments
  - Open to learning about the benefits of yoga for recovery.

- Goals:

  - Recover from injury or manage chronic pain
  - Increase flexibility and mobility
  - Gain a better understanding of how yoga can support healing.

Avatar 3, Prenatal yoga Petra

- Demographics:

  - Age: 27

- – Gender: Female
- – Occupation: Part-time teacher
- – Income: Varied.

- Psychographics:

  - – Expecting a baby and planning for pregnancy
  - – Interested in maintaining a healthy pregnancy
  - – May have limited experience with yoga, especially prenatal yoga.

- Yoga preferences:

  - – Seeks prenatal yoga classes tailored to pregnancy
  - – Values safety, comfort, and expert guidance
  - – Flexible scheduling options to accommodate pregnancy-related challenges.

- Goals:

  - – Support a healthy pregnancy
  - – Relieve pregnancy discomfort
  - – Prepare mentally and physically for childbirth.

P3 People

Yoga, by nature, is a deeply personal and transformative experience. By prioritizing the "people" element in your marketing strategy, we're aiming to co-create a personalized experience grounded in genuine, meaningful human connection. The "people" element of the Yoga for One social marketing mix is the "who" of the program story and marketing mix. As a result, it refers to all individuals who play a role in the client's experience of the program:

- *You, the yoga professional:* In the delivery of one-on-one yoga programs, your role transcends that of a simple service provider. You become the embodiment of the yoga philosophy, representing its core values, traditions, and essence. Your expertise, unique teaching style, and genuine rapport with clients influences how they are introduced to, and experience, the yoga journey. Your knowledge, teaching style, interpersonal skills, and overall demeanor significantly impact your client's experience. Being personable, understanding, and adaptable can help foster stronger relationships with your clients, leading to increased loyalty and word-of-mouth referrals.

- *The person receiving care (the client):* Understanding your clients is paramount. Recognizing their needs, preferences, limitations, and goals allows you to tailor your sessions more effectively. The better you can align your services with their individual requirements, the more valuable and satisfactory they'll find your training. Clients are looking for more than just a workout; they are seeking a holistic journey of physical, mental, and spiritual growth. The human interactions they experience throughout this journey can greatly influence their overall satisfaction and commitment to the practice.

- *Sponsoring partners:* As we aim to bring Yoga for One programs to more diverse audiences in inclusive ways, we can explore the option of partnering with sponsors of the program. In this way clients can have their yoga program partially or completely subsidized, so that it is more affordable for them. If you are engaging in such partnerships, your sponsoring partners (individuals, foundations, or organizations) become part of your "people" element in the marketing mix. Building healthy and respectful relationships with partners can have a positive impact on both our clients' outcomes and our business outcomes.

- *Supporting roles:* Anyone else involved in the client's journey to and through the program is serving in what we'll call here a supporting role. For example, if you have a friendly receptionist working at the front desk of the wellness center in which you are providing yoga services, their interaction with your clients becomes an integral part of the "people" component of the program's marketing mix. Because even small interactions can leave lasting impressions, their interaction with your clients can help to make or break the client's overall experience of the program.

P4 Product: the Yoga for One program

In a traditional marketing mix, the term "product" refers to the goods or services that a company offers to meet customer needs and wants. In the case of a one-on-one yoga program delivery, the program itself is the "what" of the program story as the product (which is actually a service). Although we will learn more in Chapters 6 and 7 about how we can co-create a one-on-one program in a way that is customized for each client, all one-on-one programs share the following key elements:

- *Personal assessment:* Before beginning any program, it's crucial to evaluate the client's physical health, flexibility, strength, and any medical concerns or limitations. This ensures that the program is safe and effective.

- *Goal setting:* Understand the client's motivations and objectives, whether it's to improve flexibility, reduce stress, enhance strength, or achieve a specific pose.

- *Customize postures for safety and alignment:* Design yoga posture (asana) sequences that cater to the client's needs and goals. Emphasize the correct alignment in every pose to prevent injuries and ensure the client reaps the maximum benefits.

- *Pranayama and practices:* Integrate pranayama (breathing exercises), meditation, mindfulness, mudras, chanting, and other practices into the sessions. These help clients to manage their energy, increase mental clarity, connect with their dharma (purpose), and experience the self-liberation of joy (aka yoga).

- *Holistic lifestyle education:* Provide education and resources on complementary practices to support the client's yoga journey and overall wellness. This can include reading materials, online tutorials, or guided meditations that they can use between sessions to enrich their practice.

- *Feedback loop:* Regularly check in with the client to gather feedback on their experience, discomfort, or any challenges faced. This continuous communication will foster trust and ensure the program remains effective.

- *Progress tracking:* Maintain a record of the client's journey, noting improvements in flexibility, strength, and mental well-being. This helps in adjusting the program as required, and provides motivation for the client.

Incorporating these ingredients will ensure that a one-on-one yoga program is comprehensive, effective, and person-centered.

P5 Price: investment of time, energy, and/or money

In any business endeavor, setting the right price for a product or service is crucial. Although we typically think about pricing in terms of financial investment (i.e., cost), I like to think of the price of a one-on-one program as the sum total of time, energy, and finances that are invested in the program by all of the people engaged in it—the yoga professional delivering it, the client receiving it, and any sponsoring and/or supporting partners helping to make it happen.

One way to approach pricing in this holistic way is to design what is commonly referred to in business as a *value ladder*. You might think of the ladder as a metaphor for the client's journey—as they grow in their awareness of and commitment to one-on-one work, they progress up the ladder. As the client ascends through their increased engagement (taken step by step), they are offered more value with increased pricing (in terms of time, energy, and/or cost).

We should note that the ladder can be constructed in an inclusive way, and with sensitivity to the social determinants of health. For example, in the case of a sponsored one-on-one yoga program, an individual client may not be paying for the program, but their investment of time and energy in the program can grow over time. In this way, their time and energy is the "price that they pay" even without financial investment. This investment of time and energy can grow and elevate over time as they progress through the client journey (aka up the value ladder).

As we can see in Figure 5, a value ladder for a Yoga for One program can be constructed to consider both the client's program journey and your time and energy commitment as a yoga professional. For example, you might create digital downloads, or on-demand videos, that can start your ideal client on the program journey—without them having to meet with you in person. In this way they can access your content with minimal investment on their part, and you can keep their financial cost low (or free) because you are not having to spend time out of your day or week meeting with each client separately. Over time, both you and they can invest in progress up the ladder. They can be invited to increase their time, energy, and financial investment as they progress through the program, and this, in turn, can contribute to the monetization (revenue generation) of your business model.

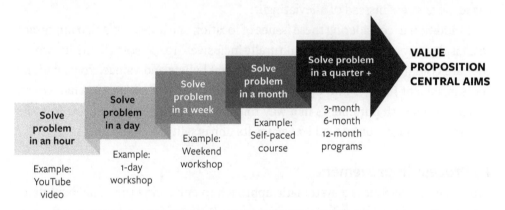

FIGURE 5: YOGA FOR ONE VALUE LADDER

Although there are many ways that you can design your one-on-one yoga program value ladder, I recommend that you co-create the ladder through engagement with your ideal clients. In this way you will be able to keep your value ladder client-centric in keeping with our social marketing approach and overarching aim to provide client-centered (person-centered) care. You can avoid over- or underpricing the value of the program, and instead support your client in their "effortless effort" as they grow in their engagement of the program in a state of ease.

P6 Place (distribution): location, access, and inclusivity

In a traditional marketing mix, the principle of "place" is typically associated with distribution in marketing terminology. Through our social marketing mix for a one-on-one yoga program, we are concerned with program location, accessibility, and inclusivity. Where can our prospective clients access the program? Where will it be delivered? How could the client's cultural identity and geographic location impact their experience of the program—favorably or unfavorably?

To illustrate the importance of place on a one-on-one yoga program, I invite you to consider how location, access, and inclusivity impact program co-creation. Imagine that you are co-creating a one-on-one yoga program through a serene yoga studio, equipped with all the essential props and ambiance. You have also received a third party grant (sponsorship) to ensure that the program is free to local first-time mothers who are experiencing financial difficulty. It sounds ideal, but is it accessible to them? Perhaps most of the new moms live far from the studio, and public transport is not available and/or affordable. Or perhaps you schedule the program at a time when they need to work. These and other concerns with regard to place can make or break the client's adoption of, and commitment to, the program. Moreover, if we don't make the program accessible by place, we could unknowingly cause more stress instead of alleviating it.

In addition to considering these issues of location and access, it is also important to consider ways that we can stay culturally inclusive—to support clients in "where they are coming from" in terms of their cultural beliefs and values. Yoga, with its roots in ancient India, is now a global phenomenon. Ideally we can do what we can to share yoga with our clients in a way that doesn't change the practice from its roots and heritage, but instead translates its universality.

P7 Process improvement

Process improvement is a systematic approach to enhancing the efficiency, effectiveness, and adaptability of processes to meet client needs or organizational goals. For a one-on-one yoga professional, refining their processes can lead to better client experiences, improved results, and more sustainable business practices. Here are several ways we can apply this "P" in the marketing mix for our one-on-one yoga program services:

- *Enhanced client experience*: Streamlined intake procedures, feedback mechanisms, and regular check-ins can lead to a smoother and more personalized experience for the client. This can increase client satisfaction and retention.

- *Better time management:* Efficient scheduling systems, timely reminders, and a structured approach to each session can ensure optimal use of time. This allows the yoga professional to possibly take on more clients, invest time in other aspects of the business, or spend less time working and more time engaging in their own quality of life.

- *Cost efficiency:* By evaluating and minimizing overheads or unnecessary expenses related to space rental, props, or marketing, a yoga professional can increase profitability.

- *Continuous learning and adaptation:* A periodic review of teaching methodologies, techniques, or curriculum can help the yoga professional stay updated and adapt to changing client needs or industry trends.

- *Increased client retention and referrals:* By regularly assessing and improving the overall client experience—from initial contact and onboarding to progress tracking and feedback management—satisfied clients are more likely to continue their lessons and recommend the teacher to others.

- *Data-driven decisions:* Implementing tools to track client progress, feedback, and session outcomes can provide valuable insights. This data can guide future program modifications and help in identifying areas of improvement.

- *Streamlined communication:* Refining communication processes, such as booking sessions, addressing queries, or sharing resources, can make interactions more effective and reduce potential misunderstandings.

- *Risk management:* A structured approach to assessing and improving processes can also identify potential risks, like physical injuries due to incorrect postures or misunderstandings due to communication gaps. Addressing these proactively can safeguard both the teacher and the client.

- *Scalability:* If a yoga teacher wishes to expand, having well-established and efficient processes makes it easier to onboard other instructors, handle more clients, or even offer group sessions without compromising on service quality.

- *Enhanced professionalism:* A systematic approach to all aspects of the business—from client interactions to session planning—exudes professionalism. This can bolster the yoga teacher's reputation and differentiate them in a competitive market.

In the case of a one-on-one yoga program, process improvement isn't just about refining your teaching or program co-creation methods. Through process improvement, you can ensure that the entire client experience is supportive for your clients and streamlined for you, as the professional.

P8 Promotion: communication and channels

In the traditional 4 Ps of the marketing mix, "promotion" refers to the set of activities, strategies, and tactics used to communicate a product's or service's features, benefits, and value to a target audience with the aim of persuading them to purchase or engage with it. Promotion serves to inform, persuade, and remind potential and existing customers about a brand, product, or service and its unique value proposition and product features. Promotion is the marketing element that focuses on creating awareness and generating demand for the offering in the market, and encompasses various tools and channels, including advertising, sales promotions, public relations, personal selling, and digital marketing. Promotion is not just about advertising a product or service; it's about establishing a dialogue with the target audience, understanding their needs, and tailoring communication to resonate with them. This is especially crucial for a one-on-one yoga program, where the client's benefits are both physical and deeply personal.

In the promotion of a one-on-one yoga program, we take an inclusive approach. Our intention is to design promotional efforts that communicate the program's value proposition in a way that is aligned with the social determinants of health—the conditions in which people are born, grow, live, work, and age. Best practices in promotional efforts aim to ensure that individuals from all backgrounds, regardless of their socio-economic status, can see the potential benefits of personalized yoga sessions for their overall health and well-being. Integrating diverse promotional channels—from traditional advertising to digital marketing and social media— ensures that the message reaches the broadest audience possible.

Best practices in messaging forums (channels)

In our social marketing approach to promoting one-on-one yoga programs, it is important that we promote the inclusive messages we design in the forums, or channels, that will deliver them to our ideal clients. Much like you need to use the right numbers on your phone to access the right channel to get your message to a friend or loved one, it's important that we think through how we are dialing in to the various promotion forums that will connect us directly to our ideal clients to promote our one-on-one yoga programs.

BUILDING AN ONLINE PRESENCE

- *Website:* Create a professional website that showcases your yoga services, qualifications, testimonials, and contact information. Optimize your website for search engines (SEO, or search engine optimization) to improve your visibility in online search results as well as for local searches by ensuring your business is listed accurately on Google My Business and other local directories. Include a blog with informative articles about yoga, health, and wellness to attract and engage visitors. After you have designed your website, invite a group of ideal customers to review it for inclusivity, efficiency, and function. In this way you can ensure that the messaging is on point, it is easy to use, and that it succeeds in helping ideal clients to register for, and engage in, your one-on-one yoga programs. You can also request reviews from satisfied clients to help build your online reputation. If you choose to do this, please be sure to ask for their explicit permission for you to do so, and have them sign a photography and video waiver that explicitly states where their likeness will be shared by you (i.e. website, brochures, etc.).

- *Social media:* Use social media platforms like Instagram, Facebook, X (formerly Twitter), and LinkedIn to share yoga-related content, photographs, and videos. Choose the social media channel/s that correspond with your ideal client. Engage with your audience by responding to comments, hosting live sessions, and sharing client success stories.

- *Online advertising:* Run online ads on platforms like Google Ads, Facebook Ads, or Instagram Ads to target specific demographics and geographic areas. Use keywords related to yoga, wellness, and your location to attract potential clients.

- *Online marketplaces:* Consider listing your services on online marketplaces such as Thumbtack or Upwork, where individuals search for various services, including yoga instruction. List your yoga services on online directories and platforms specifically designed for wellness professionals.

ENGAGING IN COMMUNITY OUTREACH AND ENGAGEMENT

Consider offering a free e-book, guide, or video series in exchange for visitors' email addresses to grow your list. Depending on your target demographic and location, consider print advertising in local magazines, newspapers, or wellness publications. Attend local wellness events, workshops, and networking groups to connect with potential clients and other professionals in the industry. Offer free or low-cost yoga classes at local community centers, schools, or libraries to introduce people to your teaching style. Volunteer to lead yoga sessions at charity events or wellness fairs to raise awareness of your services. Partner with local yoga studios, fitness centers, or gyms to offer one-on-one sessions to their members. Some studios may allow you to advertise your services within their facilities. Collaborate with other wellness practitioners, such as nutritionists or massage therapists, who may refer clients to you. Encourage your current clients to refer their friends and family to your one-on-one sessions. Establish a referral program that rewards clients for bringing in new business.

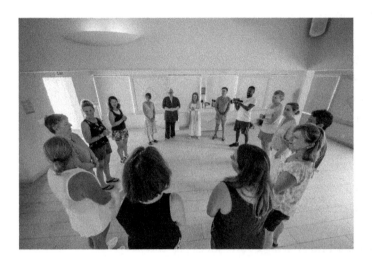

PROVIDING VALUE-IN-ADVANCE

Build an email list of interested clients and send them regular newsletters, updates, and promotions. Create a YouTube channel or use platforms like Vimeo to share yoga tutorials, tips, and advice. Include links to your website and contact information in your video descriptions.

Publish informative and valuable content on topics related to yoga and wellness on your blog or social media. Share your knowledge and establish yourself as an expert in the field. Host or participate in podcasts and webinars related to yoga and wellness to reach a broader audience and showcase your expertise.

As you can see, there are many channel options available to you to distribute your promotional messages—to prospective clients and current ones. I encourage you to choose the channels that work well for you and your clients, and don't distract you from the day-to-day demand by delivering one-on-one yoga programs. Once you determine which channels you want to focus on, you can then monitor and evaluate the performance of each channel to refine your marketing efforts over time.

Best practices in effective communication messaging

Yoga, an ancient practice that harmonizes the mind, body, and spirit, relies not just on the execution of poses but also on the connection between the instructor and the practitioner. For a yoga professional delivering one-on-one yoga programs, effective communication is paramount in ensuring that their clients achieve their physical and mental goals. Here's how you can apply effective communication practices as part of your promotional efforts in your marketing mix:

- *Active listening:* By attentively listening to clients, the yoga professional can better understand their needs, concerns, and aspirations. This allows them to tailor sessions accordingly and address specific challenges the client might be facing.

- *Empathy:* Understanding and feeling the emotions of clients allows a yoga professional to connect deeply with them. This creates a comfortable space where the client feels valued and understood, fostering a positive yoga environment.

- *Clear communication:* Clearly instructing poses, breathing techniques, and other yoga practices ensures the client's safety and maximizes the benefits of each session.

- *Open-ended questions:* By asking questions like, "How do you feel after this pose?" the yoga professional encourages clients to share their perspectives, giving the yoga professional additional insights into their experiences and needs.

- *Respect boundaries:* Recognizing and respecting physical and emotional boundaries ensures the client feels safe. This might involve asking for consent before offering a hands-on adjustment or respecting a client's wish not to delve into certain emotional or esoteric material during meditation.

- *Feedback solicitation:* Actively seeking feedback about sessions allows yoga professionals to adjust their work to the needs of the client and to improve over time. This collaborative approach helps in refining and optimizing the one-on-one yoga program.

- *Transparency:* Being open about the goals, methods, and potential challenges of the yoga journey sets realistic expectations for the client and builds trust.

- *Timely responses:* Responding to queries or concerns promptly shows clients that they are a priority, and that their well-being is of utmost importance.

- *Customized communication:* Everyone's yoga journey is unique. Tailoring communication to fit individual client needs and preferences ensures more personalized and effective sessions.

- *Education:* Educating clients about the philosophy, history, and benefits of yoga deepens their understanding and appreciation of the practice.

- *Progress updates:* Regularly updating clients on their progress keeps them motivated. Highlighting improvements can be a significant morale boost.

- *Conflict resolution:* Addressing concerns and conflicts in a calm, constructive manner helps in maintaining a harmonious trainer–client relationship.

- *Flexibility:* Being adaptable in teaching methods, communication styles, or session timings, among other things, caters to the diverse needs of clients.

- *Positive reinforcement:* Celebrating achievements, no matter how small, encourages clients to stay committed and boosts their confidence.

- *Cultural sensitivity:* Understanding and respecting cultural differences, beliefs, and practices ensures an inclusive environment where all clients feel welcomed.

- *Digital communication etiquette:* In the age of online yoga sessions and digital communication, being respectful and professional in online interactions, and understanding the nuances of digital etiquette, is crucial.

As you can see, effective communication goes beyond just imparting knowledge; it's about building connections, fostering trust, and guiding clients on a transformative journey. By incorporating these communication practices, a yoga professional can ensure that each client's yoga journey is enriching, personalized, and fulfilling.

P9 Persuasion: persuading prospectors to buy in (sales)

In the marketing of a one-on-one yoga program, sales refer to the process of persuading potential clients to invest in your services. But sales are not just about the financial transactions that occur when the client purchases your program. We are persuading them to invest more than money; we are inviting them to invest their time and energy into the program's potential. In essence we are communicating to the client the potential value of a one-on-one program generally, and our unique value proposition for its delivery specifically, so that they are persuaded to invest their time, energy, and money in the program. (In the case of third party funding, they are still investing their time and energy in the program, even if there is no financial cost.) These persuasion (sales) efforts therefore include all of the following elements:

- Client relationship building:

  - *Initial contact:* Engage with potential clients through various channels such as your website, social media, or referrals. Respond promptly to inquiries and establish a positive first impression.
  - *Active listening:* During the initial interactions, practice active listening to understand the client's goals, preferences, fitness levels, and any specific health considerations. Ask open-ended questions to gather relevant information.
  - *Personalized approach:* Tailor your communication and offerings to each client's unique needs. Highlight how your one-on-one yoga sessions can address their specific goals and challenges.

- Illuminate value and benefits:

  - *Educate clients:* Share your expertise and the benefits of one-on-one yoga sessions. Explain how personalized instruction can help clients achieve their goals more effectively compared to group classes.
  - *Highlight results:* Emphasize the potential outcomes and improvements clients can expect from your sessions, such as increased flexibility, stress reduction, pain relief, or enhanced mindfulness.
  - *Address concerns:* Be prepared to address any concerns or questions clients may have about one-on-one instruction, safety, or the yoga styles you offer.

- Customized session planning:

  - *Proposal:* Create a detailed proposal or plan for the client, outlining how the one-on-one sessions will be structured, including session frequency, duration, and goals.
  - *Demonstration:* If possible, provide a demonstration or trial session to showcase your teaching style and expertise. This allows clients to experience the benefits firsthand.
  - *Personalized benefits:* Explain how you will customize each session to the client's current abilities, goals, and any physical limitations or health considerations.

- Pricing and packages:

  - *Transparent pricing*: Clearly communicate your pricing structure, including the cost of individual sessions or packages. Ensure transparency regarding additional fees or terms.
  - *Package options*: Offer package deals or bundles that provide cost savings for clients who commit to multiple sessions. Highlight the value they will receive with investment.
  - *Payment convenience*: Set up easy and secure payment methods that allow clients to book and pay for sessions without friction.

- Overcoming objections:

  - *Address concerns*: If a client expresses concerns about pricing, scheduling, or any other aspect, address these objections professionally and provide solutions or alternatives.
  - *Benefits vs. cost*: Reinforce the benefits and value of one-on-one instruction, helping clients see that the investment is justified by the results they will achieve.

- Closing the sale:

  - *Ask for commitment*: Once the client is convinced of the value, ask for their commitment to book sessions or purchase a package. Use clear and confident language to initiate the booking process.
  - *Scheduling*: Coordinate session schedules that align with the client's availability and preferences.

- Post-sale support:

  - *Client onboarding*: After the sale, ensure a smooth onboarding process. Provide clients with all necessary information, including session logistics, preparation, and what to expect.
  - *Feedback and adjustments*: Continuously gather feedback from clients to improve your services. Be open to making adjustments to sessions or plans based on their input.
  - *Long-term relationship*: Build and nurture long-term relationships with clients by maintaining open communication, celebrating their progress, and offering incentives for continued sessions.

Effective sales for a yoga one-on-one instructor require a client-centered approach, clear communication, and a focus on delivering value. By understanding your client's needs and demonstrating how your personalized yoga instruction can help them achieve their goals, you can successfully close sales and build a thriving yoga practice.

CONCLUSION

As we have seen, you can take a conscious approach to developing your social marketing mix through what I call the 9 Ps: *presence, positioning, people, product, price, place (distribution), process (improvement), promotion,* and *persuasion.* In this way, you can co-create marketing and promotional efforts that ensure that those who need your program (prospective clients) will know about your one-on-one yoga program offerings, and understand their value enough to buy in to the promise they deliver. By meeting the client where they are in our marketing efforts, and communicating to them the potential value our work together offers, we can begin a healthy and inclusive relationship with our clients, before we have met them! This relationship sets the state for our direct work with clients, which we will explore next.

CHAPTER 5

Meeting the Client Where They Are

ASSESSMENT TOOLS

In the co-creation of a one-on-one yoga program, we aim to take an inclusive and evidence-informed approach to personalize a yoga program for the unique needs and goals of the individual client. In this chapter, we will explore how we can begin the program co-creation process through the evaluation practices of the client intake, interview, and asana assessment. You'll discover how you can carry forward what you learn about the client through these assessment practices in Chapters 6 and 7 (where we'll discuss evidence-informed program planning and inclusive practice design).

EVALUATION VS. ASSESSMENT

In our one-on-one yoga program approach, the program plan is the road map of where we are going; it is how we get from where we are to where we want to be. In Chapter 6, you will learn how you can design the program as your road map. In this chapter, we will explore how you can build the GPS that will help you navigate the map and the journey—through the practices of evaluation (GPS) and assessment (location).

The practices of assessment and evaluation work together to ensure that a one-on-one yoga program stays aligned with the needs and goals of the client. Operating together, they support our aims to provide person-centered programs for our clients that are both effective and relevant. As a practice, *assessment* is a process that primarily focuses on gathering information so we can accurately understand the client's current condition/s, challenges, and concern/s. You might think of assessment as a form of geo-locating because it gives us an idea of the client's current location (state) of well-being needs, challenges, and goals. The process of examining assessments over time, while monitoring how the client is progressing towards their goals, is referred to as *evaluation*.

Essential components of the evaluation process include tracking progress in areas identified during the pre-planning phase, gathering feedback to understand the client's perceptions of the program, and regularly revisiting the initial objectives to ensure they're being met. Through assessment, we understand more about where the client is, and isn't, relative to their goal (destination). Through evaluation, we understand why that matters, and we can adjust what we will do next to get us back on track to our goals (where we are going).

OUR EVALUATION AND ASSESSMENT FRAMEWORK: THE KOSHA THEORETICAL MODEL

As you may know from your own yoga training journey, the kosha system framework is believed to date back to the *Upanishads*. The term "kosha" is synonymous with the terms "sheath" and "layer." Each kosha represents a different dimension or layer of the human being, providing a framework to understand the holistic nature of an individual. There are typically five koshas, although some traditions may describe more or fewer layers. Much like the socio-ecological model that we reviewed in Chapter 2, the kosha model is also a systems model. This means that when one layer (kosha) is impacted, positively or negatively, all of the layers are impacted through a ripple effect.

There are five primary koshas. For our one-on-one yoga program approach to evaluation and assessment, we will focus our attention on the five primary koshas. Although we will review these sheaths separately, they are conceptually integrated. In other words, they are not "rings" around the soul of an individual; they are different dimensions of an individual that are simultaneously part of that individual's being.

- *Annamaya kosha (physical sheath)*: Representing the physical body, the anna-maya kosha encompasses the physical aspects of the Self, including the muscles, bones, organs, and skin. It is associated with the physical sensations and experiences of the body. It is also referred to as the food sheath, and it refers to not only the real food we take in for nutrition, but all of the "food" we take in during the day. Our environment impacts us; we are part of nature and it impacts us as much as we impact it. Our asana practice is often associated with this sheath, but there are many other practices we can use to help us manage it. This layer is what I like to think of as our human performance system; it is the ecosystem of our human physiology, which is impacted by, and impacts, the other layers of Self.

- *Pranamaya kosha (vital energy sheath):* This layer is related to the body's vital energy or life force, often referred to as prana and/or vayus. It involves the breath, circulation, and the energy flows within the body, and the chakra system is conceptualized to live here as well. The pranamaya kosha is associated with the breath and the subtle life force that animates the physical body. In contemporary terms, this layer is one that closely relates to our "social battery"—how much energy or vitality we do or don't have to engage in the world. Pranayama practices, mudras, mantras, and chanting can help us to regulate this sheath, as can certain asanas (postures). Through active engagement of the bandhas, we are connecting the annamaya and pranamaya layers, activating our life force while removing the granthis (blocks) to our vitality.

- *Manomaya kosha (mental sheath):* This sheath pertains to the mind and mental processes, and includes thoughts, emotions, desires, and the cognitive functions of the brain. The manomaya kosha represents the layer of the Self that interacts with the external world through thoughts and feelings, and we can think of this layer as mostly related to our human "ego" mind. Here we have the full spectrum of our humanity—with thoughts and feelings that we can sometimes manage and other times get away from us. The practices of mindfulness, meditation, and yoga nidra (yogic sleep) can help us to regulate this sheath, and to build a capacity for regulating our emotions over time when life's plot twists present themselves.

- *Vijnanamaya kosha (wisdom sheath):* This layer is associated with higher intellect, intuition, wisdom, and discernment. It represents our ability to make decisions, exercise judgment, and gain deeper insight into ourselves and the world. In my applied research and one-on-one work with clients, I think of this layer as being closely connected to our life story—and whether or not we feel like we are living the life we want to live and are meant to live. As we go deeply into this layer of our Self, we are able to witness our Self without judgment and with acceptance—celebrating our unique individual gifts and the dharma (calling) of our life's purpose.

- *Anandamaya kosha (bliss sheath):* The innermost layer represents a state of bliss and profound joy. It is often described as the true essence or core of an individual, where the individual experiences a sense of unity and oneness with the universe. This layer is believed to be the source of deep inner peace and spiritual realization, and our connection to a force (Source) that is greater than ourselves. Here we connect to the light of our common humanity, and to the spiritual well-spring of God.

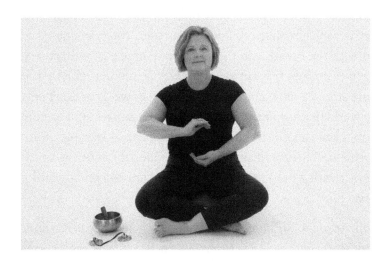

OUR APPROACH TO EVALUATION AND ASSESSMENT: THE YOGA FOR ONE SOAP PROCESS

The SOAP framework, which stands for Subjective, Objective, Assessment, and Plan, originated in the medical field as a standardized approach to documenting patient information and managing patient care. The acronym "SOAP" has historically been a way to organize individual patient encounters. Each component of the SOAP process is intended to capture a specific type of information:

- *Subjective:* The patient's reported symptoms or complaints.

- *Objective:* The tangible, measurable data such as physical examination findings, lab results, and vital signs.

- *Assessment:* The healthcare provider's interpretation of the patient's current condition.

- *Plan:* The proposed treatment or next steps for the patient's care.

Over the years, the SOAP process has transcended the boundaries of medicine so that it is now incorporated into many other health disciplines, including nursing, physical therapy, mental health, and complementary therapies like chiropractic and yoga therapy. Its adaptability and structured approach have made it a valuable tool for professionals seeking a consistent method to document and share client or patient information.

In the co-creation of a one-on-one yoga program, I have adapted the SOAP process to keep the process of evaluation and assessment manageable for the yoga professional and user-friendly for the client. You can apply this approach or adapt it based on your preferences and your client's needs:

- *Subjective:* In this phase we review the client's intake form, and gather information (through the client's intake form and waivers) to gain a better understanding of the client's health situation and medical concerns, current state of well-being, lifestyle behaviors, doshas, and gunas. We also actively listen as the client shares their lived experience during the client interview, to learn more about their story. In this way, this phase enables us to better understand the first "E" of our evidence-informed practice model: the lived *experience* of the client.

- *Objective:* In this phase we apply the other two "Es" of evidence-informed practice (our *expertise* and *evidence*). We apply our expertise in the witnessing of the client's story and situation, and note what we objectively see through healthcare and/or public health points of view (depending on our scope of practice). We review the evidence the client presents to us (through the data they share in their intake form/s and interview) as well as the evidence basis we can find in the empirical research (i.e., the evidence base). By combining insights from our own expertise and professional field with evidence collected from the client and the latest research, we are able to get a 360-degree view of the client, while contextualizing their subjective lived experience with our informed objectivity.

- *Assessment:* In this phase we reflect on what we know about the client's current priorities and future goals, and then assess whether or not a referral is needed before we work with the client. If the client is cleared to proceed (and referrals are not necessary), we can then assess whether or not a one-on-one yoga program intervention is in alignment with the client's needs and goals, and whether or not we are the best yoga professional for the client to work with. Here we also assess (through the practice of shared decision-making) which kosha we feel is emerging as an area of priority, and then decide if we want to engage in further assessment of that kosha. For example, we may find that we want to focus on annamaya kosha; however, we may realize we need to assess the client moving in asanas before we go into designing a program based on optimizing this kosha.

- *Plan:* This prioritization process and continued assessments flow well into the final phase of the SOAP process—planning. In Chapter 6, you'll see how you can use my one-on-one yoga program logic model template to co-create a program plan with the client—to help them to go from where they are today (their priorities) to where they want to be tomorrow (their vision of program success).

The five action steps of SOAP

As you can see, we are viewing SOAP as more than a record-keeping strategy, but instead as our approach to evaluation and assessment. In my work with one-on-one clients I have developed a five-step process for moving through these four phases of SOAP in a user-friendly and logical manner:

- Step 1: Consent forms and waivers

- Step 2: Integrative health history

- Step 3: The client interview

- Step 4: Asana assessment session

- Step 5: Program and practice plan

In this chapter, we will discuss steps 1 through 4. Then, in Chapter 6 we will discuss how to go about the fifth step—planning out the program plan (for yoga on and off the mat).

STEP 1: CONSENT FORMS AND WAIVERS

Every yoga session and program has its own inherent risks. Consent forms and waivers play vital roles in ensuring clients are aware of these risks and assume responsibility for their participation. This legal documentation ensures that both the yoga professional and client are protected while serving as an important step in the boundary-setting process of client relationship building.

In the context of a one-on-one yoga program, it is important to ensure that clients' boundaries are protected and respected, as well as yoga professionals' boundaries. The consent process occurs when both the client and the yoga professional have a clear understanding of what a program, practice session, or pose involves—before they experience it—and mutually agree to proceed. For example, before starting a one-on-one yoga program, a yoga professional may be required by their professional insurance to request that all clients sign initial participation waivers. By signing a waiver, clients acknowledge that they are willing to accept the inherent risks of beginning a yoga program. They also acknowledge that they are aware of potential mishaps, however rare they might be.

For the yoga professional, a waiver acts as a protective shield against potential legal claims arising from unforeseen injuries. But for a waiver to be effective, it must be comprehensive, detailing potential risks, ensuring client understanding, and clearly stating that the client cannot sue the yoga professional in the event of an injury. Waivers are best developed by legal counsel so that they serve to protect everyone's legal rights and do not inadvertently cause legal harm. Keeping these signed waivers stored safely is an important legal practice too.

In addition to program-level consent, it is also important for yoga professionals to request consent before asking clients to engage in new postures and/or practices. For example, the yoga professional may ask for permission before adjusting the client's posture, especially in the case of hands-on adjustments. Please remember that hands-on adjustments are a professional skill in need of adequate training; it is legally risky and professionally problematic to engage in hands-on adjustments without the proper training to do so.

It is important to note that both consent forms and waivers are not only legal documents; they are also professionally connected to our scope of practice through insurance coverage. Most insurance policies cover us for operating in our scope of practice, in the yoga professional credentials we have obtained. If we step outside of our scope of practice and/or our clients do not sign waivers and consent forms, we may jeopardize our insurance coverage. Please be sure to check your insurance policies and check in with your insurance carrier as well as your legal counsel to ensure that all consent forms, waivers, and insurance policies are in alignment—to protect you and your client in a one-on-one yoga program.

It is imperative for yoga professionals to consult with insurance professionals to tailor the best protection plan, which will usually include general liability insurance, professional practice insurance, and business insurance. If you are operating a studio within your home, you'll also need to ensure that your studio insurance coverage and homeowners' insurance are in alignment, and that both insurance carriers acknowledge their awareness that you are operating a business in your home. (*Author's note:* Please do not misconstrue this section as insurance advice, and please be sure to check with your legal and insurance partners for the guidance that is best for you and your business.)

STEP 2: INTEGRATIVE HEALTH HISTORY

A comprehensive understanding of a client's health history, including medical conditions, past injuries, and any advice they've been given, is vital. It allows the yoga professional to understand potential reactions—even in practices considered moderate, like mantras or mudras. This ensures that each session is tailored to be safe and beneficial for the client, maximizing the therapeutic potential of yoga. Through the intake of the client's health history, we get a snapshot of the client's quality of life, lifestyle medicine behaviors, and health challenges.

As we engage in this process, it is important for us to have an awareness of the complexities surrounding health information data collection and privacy management. Although every yoga professional operates in a unique locality, with its own local, regional, and national policies, I would like to offer here some general areas for your consideration (or "things to think about") with regard to health history data collection.

Privacy management: the Health Insurance Portability and Accountability Act (HIPAA)

In the United States, licensed health professionals are bound to adhere to HIPAA. HIPAA is a US law designed to provide privacy standards to protect patients' medical records and other health information provided to health plans, doctors, hospitals, and other healthcare providers. Because most yoga professionals do not operate as licensed health providers (unless they have another allied health credential), they are not legally bound to follow HIPAA policies. However, we have the option of following these guidelines, whether or not we are required to do so.

The majority (although not all) of the HIPAA guidelines can help yoga professionals to consider how we handle and protect our client's personal health information. Establishing trust with clients means ensuring their information remains private and secure. Whether or not you are compelled to follow HIPAA guidance (or other health information policies in your country), I encourage you to also consult with a legal professional to ensure you can protect yourself and your business from legal harm from a privacy and data management perspective. In addition to following specific guidance you receive from your practice field policies and your personal attorney, here are some general best practices that you can follow:

- *Privacy of health information:* If you receive any health information from your clients, such as medical histories or specific health conditions, it's important to keep this information confidential. This applies particularly if you're working in a healthcare setting like a rehab center or hospital.

- *Secure storage and handling:* Any health information you record should be stored securely and shared only with those who need to know for the client's care. This includes both digital and physical records.

- *Permission to share information:* If you need to share a client's health information with other professionals (like doctors or therapists), you must get explicit consent from the client, unless it's for standard healthcare operations.

- *Limited access:* Only provide the minimum necessary information when it's required for a specific purpose. Avoid sharing more than what is needed.

- *Training and policies:* If you are part of a larger organization, such as a hospital or wellness center, they likely have HIPAA training and policies. Make sure you're familiar with these and follow them strictly.

- *Breach notification:* In case of any breach of private health information, there are specific protocols to follow, which usually involve notifying the affected individuals and possibly federal agencies.

Let's remember, HIPAA compliance is required for licensed healthcare providers, insurers, and certain health administrators, and is usually optional for yoga professionals who are not licensed. Whether or not compliance is required, maintaining client confidentiality and privacy is a good practice in any health-related profession.

Integrative health history

Because yoga is a practice of integrative health and holism, client intake forms aim to be comprehensive. However, it is important that we are also not exhausting—both the client and ourselves—with an intake form that is too long. In an effort to provide you with a menu of options for your own health history forms, I am sharing here the client intake information I request from new clients. Feel free to pull down from this list a shorter health history and/or to embellish it with additional surveys—depending on your unique situation. Keep in mind you'll want to be sure that your legal and insurance professional team will want to approve your final forms, and that these are provided here for educational purposes only.

"Menu" of options for the client intake form

My integrative health history form requests information that is relevant to both healthcare and public health points of view, and requests both biomedical and Ayurvedic information. As noted, you are encouraged to only request data that is relevant to your scope of practice, and to have your legal and insurance team review your form and collection process to be sure to protect you and your business from further liability.

General Information

The following *Integrative Health History Form* aims to capture the important information for client assessment in a one-on-one yoga program. You are invited to adapt the survey for your purposes, and to adjust the questions based on your unique program niche and client goals. Please remember to share your final survey with your legal and insurance team to ensure that you are operating within your scope of practice, with low risk. And, please remember to keep all data collected in a safe and secure place, to protect client privacy and confidentiality.

INTEGRATIVE HEALTH HISTORY

Personal information

Name: ....

Age: ....

How do you identify your gender: ....

Contact information (City/State/Zip/Phone/Email): ....

....

....

Emergency contact information: ....

May we contact you via text?   ☐ Yes   ☐ No

May we contact you via email? ☐ Yes   ☐ No

Medical condition

How would you describe your overall medical condition?

☐ Excellent
☐ Good
☐ Average
☐ Poor

Do you have any current or past injuries? If yes, please specify.

☐ Yes: ....
☐ No

Are you currently on any medication or undergoing medical treatment? If yes, please specify.

☐ Yes: ....
☐ No

Yoga experience

How familiar are you with yoga practices?

- ☐ Beginner (never practiced or only a few times)
- ☐ Explorer (have practiced <6 months)
- ☐ Practitioner (practice regularly >6 months)
- ☐ Yoga professional (Circle all that apply: Yoga Coach, Yoga Teacher, Yoga Therapist, Allied Health Professional)

What are your primary goals for this yoga program? . . . .
(Examples: flexibility, strength, relaxation, posture, stress reduction, wellness, quality of life)

If you have practiced yoga previously, what did you like and/or dislike about it?

. . . .

If you have not practiced yoga previously, what led you to decide to give it a try?

. . . .

Overall comfort and limitations

Are there specific yoga poses or practices you find challenging or uncomfortable? If yes, please specify.

- ☐ Yes: . . . .
- ☐ No

Additional information

Are there any other concerns, preferences, or information you'd like to share regarding your physical well-being or expectations for this yoga program?

. . . .

WHO-5

The WHO-5 is a well-being survey instrument which helps us to understand your current state of well-being[18].

Please indicate for each of the five statements which is closest to how you have been feeling over the last two weeks. Notice that higher numbers mean better well-being.

5 = All of the time
4 = Most of the time
3 = More than half of the time
2 = Less than half of the time
1 = Some of the time
0 = At no time

Over the last two weeks:	All of the time	Most of the time	More than half of the time	Less than half of the time	Some of the time	At no time
1. I have felt cheerful and in good spirits	5	4	3	2	1	O
2. I have felt calm and relaxed	5	4	3	2	1	O
3. I have felt active and vigorous	5	4	3	2	1	O
4. I woke up feeling refreshed and rested	5	4	3	2	1	O
5. My daily life has been filled with things that interest me	5	4	3	2	1	O

WHO-5 inclusivity recommendations

After the client has completed the survey, we can review both their responses to each question and their composite score. Although this survey was not originally designed for this purpose, in the practice field I use each question as an indicator (or initial screening) for each of the koshas.

"I have felt cheerful and in good spirits."

This question tells me more about their overall emotional well-being and their anandamaya kosha. If this score is 1 or 2, then this would indicate that this is a kosha that we can focus on improving for the Yoga for One program.

"I have felt calm and relaxed."

This question tells me more about their mental well-being and their manomaya kosha. If this score is 1 or 2, then this would indicate that this is a kosha that we can focus on improving for the Yoga for One program.

"I have felt active and vigorous."

This question tells me more about their physical well-being: annamaya kosha. If this score is 1 or 2, then this would indicate that this is a kosha that we can focus on improving for the Yoga for One program.

"I woke up feeling refreshed and rested."

This question tells me more about their social well-being, their overall energy level and their pranamaya kosha. If this score is 1 or 2, then this would indicate that this is a kosha that we can focus on improving for the Yoga for One program.

"My daily life has been filled with things that interest me."

This question tells me more about their purpose well-being and their vijnanamaya kosha. If this score is 1 or 2, then this would indicate that this is a kosha that we can focus on improving for the Yoga for One program.

In addition to these insights gained from each question on the WHO-5, we can also learn more about the client by their total composite score. According to the tool guidelines, the total score is multiplied by 4, with a total possible score of 100. For clients that score a 50 or lower, a referral for further depression screening is recommended. This means that those with a composite score of 50 or less should be referred to an allied health professional trained in mental health assessment, specifically in depression assessment. Keep in mind the low WHO-5 score does not necessarily mean they have depression; this is why further depression testing is warranted. If we do find ourselves in the situation that the client has a low score (and is in need of a referral), my suggestion is to share this with them carefully, and compassionately. For example, we might say, "I wanted to take a moment to talk with you about your recent assessment. Your WHO-5 well-being score is indicating that 'further inquiry needed'. What that means is that the survey is telling us that you would benefit from a more in-depth mental health screening—one that is more in-depth than this simple 5-question survey. I want to reassure you that this result is common, and doesn't necessarily mean that anything is wrong at this time. It simply means that further information is needed to ensure you receive the best support possible for your well-being. A mental health professional is trained to offer these in-depth screenings, and to provide you with valuable insights and resources tailored to your needs."

Dosha assessment (vata, pitta, kapha)

Rooted in ancient Indian healing traditions, Ayurveda believes that understanding someone's unique dosha is key to achieving optimal well-being. Doshas describe our general constitution, which is formed by the five elements—earth, water, fire, air, and ether. By discovering our dominant dosha or doshas, we can better align our lifestyle, diet, and activities with our intrinsic nature, promoting harmony, health, and vitality. Each individual has a unique dosha constitution, known as their Prakriti, which is determined at the time of birth and remains relatively stable throughout life. Imbalances in the doshas, known as Vikriti, can occur due to lifestyle, diet, and environmental factors, and can lead to various health issues.

DOSHA SCREENING SURVEY

This survey is designed to provide insights into your dominant dosha based on various physical and behavioral characteristics. Answer each section authentically to unveil a more profound understanding of yourself through the lens of Ayurveda. And please remember that everyone has all three doshas.

Body type: *Choose one*

☐ Slim or slender [1 point vata]
☐ Medium build [1 point pitta]
☐ Stocky or well-built [1 point kapha]

Skin type: *Choose one*

☐ Dry, rough, or cold [1 point vata]
☐ Warm, reddish, or prone to acne [1 point pitta]
☐ Smooth, moist, or oily [1 point kapha]

Hair type: *Choose one*

☐ Dry or frizzy [1 point vata]
☐ Fine, straight, reddish, or prematurely graying [1 point pitta]
☐ Thick, wavy, or oily [1 point kapha]

Temperament: *Choose all that apply*

☐ Creative, quick to learn and forget [1 point vata]
☐ Intelligent, focused, organized [1 point pitta]
☐ Calm, slow to learn and forget [1 point kapha]

Emotional response to stress: *Choose all that apply*

☐ Anxiety or fear [1 point vata]
☐ Irritability or anger [1 point pitta]
☐ Withdrawal or attachment [1 point kapha]

Activity level: *Choose all that apply*

☐ Active and restless [1 point vata]
☐ Moderate activity level with purposefulness [1 point pitta]
☐ Slow, steady, and resistant to change [1 point kapha]

Appetite: *Choose all that apply*

☐ Variable, often skipping meals [1 point vata]
☐ Strong, gets irritable if missed a meal [1 point pitta]
☐ Steady but can easily skip meals without discomfort [1 point kapha]

Preferences: *Choose all that apply*

☐ Prefers warm, salty, or sour foods [1 point vata]
☐ Prefers cool, sweet, bitter, or astringent foods [1 point pitta]
☐ Prefers dry, warm, or pungent foods [1 point kapha]

Scoring for doshas

Total vata: . . . . /8

Total pitta: . . . . /8

Total kapha: . . . . /8

Dosha inclusivity recommendations

In a personalized yoga program, recognizing these doshas helps in customizing practices to promote balance, well-being, and personal growth. Let's explore each dosha from a balanced vs. imbalanced perspective, through the lens of the koshas. Through this understanding, we can determine if further kosha-based screenings, assessments, and/or referrals are needed.

VATA (AIR AND ETHER) IN BALANCE

Vata-dominant types are usually creative, active, and energetic; they fly with the winds of change. Vata-dominant types have energy that is dynamic and ever changing, and may benefit from yoga programs that are grounding and stabilizing, helping them to balance out any excess air and ether elements and to center their active minds.

VATA OUT OF BALANCE

An allied health referral may be indicated with the signs of vata imbalance shown in Table 2. Vata governs movement, communication, and the nervous system. When vata-dominant types find themselves out of balance, they can experience changes in any or all of their koshas, as noted. Depending on the severity of the issue, another screening may be needed or a direct referral may be warranted. When in doubt, refer.

PITTA (FIRE AND WATER) IN BALANCE

Pitta types are often intelligent, goal-oriented, and leadership-driven; they are the most prone for burnout. They may benefit from a yoga program that provides soothing and cooling experiences to balance out their fiery nature and to recharge their batteries.

PITTA OUT OF BALANCE

Pitta governs metabolism, digestion, and transformation in the body. When pitta is out of balance, it can impact any or all of their koshas, as noted in Table 2. Depending on the severity of the issue, another screening may be needed or a direct referral may be warranted. When in doubt, refer.

KAPHA (EARTH AND WATER) IN BALANCE

Kapha types tend to be calm, grounded, and reliable. Kapha-dominant people possess a steady and nurturing energy. Yoga sessions might focus on stimulating and invigorating practices to balance the earth and water elements predominant in kapha.

KAPHA OUT OF BALANCE

Kapha governs stability, structure, and lubrication in the body. When kapha is out of balance, it can impact any or all of their koshas, as noted in Table 2. Depending on the severity of the issue, another screening may be needed or a direct referral may be warranted.

VATA–PITTA OR PITTA–VATA

Some people are dominant in both vata and pitta qualities if they score 5 or more in more than one category; they are creative and goal-oriented. They may also have a combination of challenges (imbalances) from both categories. Their yoga programs can focus on a mix of grounding and cooling techniques. Incorporating both calming and moderate-intensity postures can help in balancing these doshas.

PITTA–KAPHA OR KAPHA–PITTA

Some people are dominant in both kapha and pitta qualities; they are intelligent and grounded. They may also have a combination of challenges (imbalances) from both categories. Their yoga programs can interweave invigorating practices to counter kapha's sluggishness with cooling techniques to pacify pitta's heat.

KAPHA–VATA OR VATA–KAPHA

Some people are dominant in both kapha and vata; they are creative and grounded. Their yoga programs can focus on both stimulation and grounding. A combination of dynamic sequences and restorative postures can be ideal.

Table 2: Vata, pitta, and kapha imbalances in the koshas

Annamaya kosha		
Vata imbalance	Pitta imbalance	Kapha imbalance
Digestive issues: Irregular bowel movements, including constipation, gas, bloating, and dry stools; sensitivity to certain foods, leading to digestive discomfort	*Digestive issues:* Hyperacidity, acid reflux, or heartburn; frequent loose stools or diarrhea; a strong craving for spicy, sour, or hot foods	*Weight gain:* Unexplained weight gain, often associated with slow metabolism; difficulty losing weight despite efforts to do so
Joint and muscle pain: Aches and pains in the joints and muscles; stiffness, especially in the morning or in cold weather	*Skin problems:* Inflammatory skin conditions such as acne, rosacea, or hives; excessive sweating, especially with an offensive odor; sensitivity to sunlight, leading to sunburn	*Congestion and mucus:* Frequent nasal congestion or sinus issues; excessive mucus production, leading to conditions like colds, coughs, or allergies

cont.

Annamaya kosha		
Vata imbalance	**Pitta imbalance**	**Kapha imbalance**
Dry skin and hair: Dry, rough, or flaky skin; brittle nails and hair; dry and cracked lips	*Inflammation:* Inflammatory conditions such as gastritis, colitis, or tendonitis; swelling and redness in joints or other body parts	*Slow digestion:* Slow and sluggish digestion; feelings of fullness and heaviness after eating, even with small meals
Irregular menstrual cycles: Irregular periods or changes in menstrual flow; increased menstrual pain or discomfort	*Excessive heat:* Feeling excessively hot, especially at night; night sweats	*Oily skin and hair:* Excessive oiliness of the skin and scalp; greasy hair and frequent acne outbreaks
Dryness in the body: Dry eyes, mouth, and throat; excessive thirst	*Strong appetite and digestion:* A consistently strong appetite; rapid digestion, often feeling hungry shortly after eating.	*Water retention:* Swelling or puffiness in the body, especially in the hands, feet, and face; edema or retention of excess fluids
Sensitivity to cold weather: Feeling excessively cold, even in mild weather; cold extremities, such as cold hands and feet	*Yellowish skin or eyes:* Yellowing of the skin or eyes, indicating potential liver or gallbladder involvement	*Aversion to cold and dampness:* Feeling cold and damp, especially in humid or rainy weather; a preference for warm and dry environments
Weight loss: Unintended weight loss due to a fast metabolism and poor absorption of nutrients	*Hormonal imbalances:* Irregular menstrual cycles or heavy menstruation; hormonal acne or other skin issues related to hormonal fluctuations	

Pranamaya kosha		
Vata imbalance	**Pitta imbalance**	**Kapha imbalance**
Fatigue: Low energy levels, especially in the afternoon; feeling easily fatigued and overwhelmed	*Sleep disturbances:* Difficulty falling asleep due to an active mind; frequent nightmares or vivid dreams	*Lethargy and fatigue:* Persistent feelings of lethargy and heaviness; difficulty getting motivated or feeling sluggish throughout the day
Insomnia: Difficulty falling asleep or staying asleep; restless or light sleep with frequent awakenings	*Vision problems:* Eye conditions such as redness, inflammation, or sensitivity to light	*Excessive sleep:* Long and deep sleep patterns; difficulty waking up in the morning

Manomaya kosha		
Vata imbalance	**Pitta imbalance**	**Kapha imbalance**
Anxiety and nervousness: Heightened anxiety, nervousness, or excessive worrying; racing thoughts and an inability to relax	*Irritability and anger:* Increased irritability, impatience, and a short temper; frequent outbursts of anger or frustration	*Depression:* A tendency towards depression or a lack of enthusiasm; emotional heaviness and sadness

		Slow speech and thought: Slow, deliberate speech and thought processes; difficulty making decisions quickly
Vijnanamaya kosha		
Vata imbalance	Pitta imbalance	Kapha imbalance
Poor concentration: Difficulty focusing and staying on task; forgetfulness and mental fog	*Competitive nature*: An intense desire to excel and compete, sometimes at the expense of others; a tendency to overwork or push oneself too hard	*Stubbornness and resistance to change*: Resistance to change and difficulty adapting to new circumstances; a preference for routine and familiarity
Anandamaya kosha		
Vata imbalance	Pitta imbalance	Kapha imbalance
Mood swings: Frequent mood swings, ranging from excitement to anxiety and fear; emotional instability and difficulty handling stress	*Strong perfectionist tendencies*: An overwhelming need for perfection and control; being overly critical of oneself and others	*Attachment*: Strong attachment to possessions, people, or routines; difficulty letting go of old habits or belongings

Trigunas survey (sattva, rajas, tamas): qualities

In the practices of yoga and Ayurveda, the trigunas—sattva (purity, harmony, illumination), rajas (activity, passion), and tamas (inertia, darkness)—represent the three fundamental energies that govern our human experience. These are qualities or attributes that describe the "states" or "tendencies" of an individual. While gunas are more subtle than doshas, they give us insights into our innate nature and tendencies, thereby paving the way for personal growth, harmony, and well-being. Our experience of the gunas changes over time due to life circumstances and personal growth.

TRIGUNA SCREENING SURVEY

This survey explores your general tendencies or "general ways of being", that are known as the trigunas. Answer each section with honesty and self-reflection. When in doubt about a particular response, go with the response that is more common or frequent than the others.

Mind state

- ☐ Calm, peaceful, clear [1 point sattva]
- ☐ Restless, desiring, agitated [1 point rajas]
- ☐ Dull, lethargic, confused [1 point tamas]

Reaction to challenges

- ☐ Reflective, seeks understanding [1 point sattva]
- ☐ Active, seeks solutions quickly [1 point rajas]
- ☐ Avoidant, feels overwhelmed [1 point tamas]

Learning style

- ☐ Grasps concepts clearly, enjoys contemplation [1 point sattva]
- ☐ Fast learner, but can be easily distracted [1 point rajas]
- ☐ Slow to learn, needs repetition [1 point tamas]

Activity level

- ☐ Balanced, purposeful activity [1 point sattva]
- ☐ Constant activity, often without rest [1 point rajas]
- ☐ Inactive, prefers rest and sleep [1 point tamas]

Dietary habits

- ☐ Prefers fresh, wholesome, and nourishing foods [1 point sattva]
- ☐ Attracted to spicy, salty, or stimulating foods [1 point rajas]
- ☐ Prefers heavy, stale, or overprocessed foods [1 point tamas]

Sleep patterns

☐ Regular, restful sleep of about 7–8 hours [1 point sattva]
☐ Interrupted sleep, often with vivid dreams [1 point rajas]
☐ Deep, prolonged sleep, often more than 9 hours [1 point tamas]

Communication style

☐ Clear, truthful, and uplifting [1 point sattva]
☐ Energetic, can sometimes be argumentative [1 point rajas]
☐ Slow, reserved, or often unresponsive [1 point tamas]

Conflict resolution

☐ Seeks understanding and harmony [1 point sattva]
☐ Can be confrontational, driven by a need to "win" [1 point rajas]
☐ Avoids conflict, can be passive-aggressive [1 point tamas]

Scoring for gunas

Total sattva: . . . . /8

Total rajas: . . . . /8

Total tamas: . . . . /8

Guna inclusivity recommendations

In a personalized yoga program, the gunas help us to understand the overall tendencies, or qualities, of the human. Let's explore what each triguna looks like from a balanced vs. imbalanced perspective, through the lens of the koshas. Through this understanding, we can determine if further kosha-based screenings, assessments, and/or referrals are needed.

SATTVA (PURITY, HARMONY, ILLUMINATION) IN BALANCE

Sattva is the quality of balance, harmony, purity, and calmness. When we are in balance, we are in a peaceful yet dynamic state of equilibrium between rajas and tamas.

SATTVA OUT OF BALANCE

- When sattva is out of balance, it can impact any or all of their koshas. Depending on the severity of the issue, another screening may be needed or a direct referral may be warranted. When in doubt, refer.

- *Annamaya kosha sattva imbalance:* Sattva imbalance can manifest in the physical body as a sense of discomfort or disconnection. An individual may experience physical symptoms such as lethargy, digestive issues, or even psychosomatic ailments.

- *Pranamaya kosha sattva imbalance:* Prana, or life force energy, flows more smoothly when sattva is in balance. An imbalance in sattva can lead to disruptions in prana flow, which may result in reduced vitality, energy stagnation, or fluctuations in the breath.

- *Manomaya kosha sattva imbalance:* Sattva is closely associated with mental clarity and purity. When sattva is imbalanced, the mind may become clouded with negative thoughts, emotions, and restlessness. An individual may experience increased mental agitation, anxiety, or confusion.

- *Vijnanamaya kosha sattva imbalance:* The wisdom sheath represents higher knowledge and intuitive wisdom. When sattva is out of balance, an individual's ability to access and trust their inner wisdom may be compromised. This can lead to difficulty in making clear decisions and discerning the truth.

- *Anandamaya kosha sattva imbalance:* Sattva plays a pivotal role in experiencing inner peace and bliss. An imbalance in sattva can lead to a sense of inner turmoil, discontent, and an inability to connect with the inherent bliss that exists within each individual.

RAJAS (ACTIVITY, PASSION)

- This quality represents activity, change, passion, and dynamism. An individual dominated by rajas might be restless, overly active, or anxious. The yoga program for them can be designed to help calm and ground their energies.

- *Annamaya kosha rajas imbalance:* An imbalance in rajas can manifest in the physical body as excess energy and restlessness. This can lead to issues such as insomnia, overexertion, and a tendency to push the body beyond its limits.

- *Pranamaya kosha rajas imbalance:* Rajas can disrupt the flow of prana, the life force energy, leading to irregularities in energy levels. An individual may experience periods of hyperactivity and then sudden crashes in energy.

- *Manomaya kosha rajas imbalance:* The mental sheath is particularly influenced by rajas. An imbalance in rajas can result in an overactive mind filled with racing thoughts, desires, and attachments. This can lead to mental agitation, anxiety, and difficulty in finding mental calm.

- *Vijnanamaya kosha rajas imbalance:* When rajas is dominant, it can cloud judgment and prevent clear discernment. An individual may find it challenging to access their inner wisdom and make well-informed decisions.

- *Anandamaya kosha rajas imbalance:* Rajas can disrupt the experience of inner peace and bliss. Instead of contentment and fulfillment, an individual may constantly seek external stimuli and pleasures, leading to temporary highs followed by crashes and dissatisfaction.

TAMAS (INERTIA, DARKNESS)

- This quality signifies darkness, inertia, laziness, and delusion. Someone showing a tamasic nature might feel lazy, lethargic, or even depressed. The yoga routine should be invigorating and energizing to rouse them from this inertia.

- *Annamaya kosha tamas imbalance:* An imbalance in tamas can manifest in the physical body as sluggishness and lethargy. Individuals may experience chronic fatigue, low energy levels, and a lack of motivation to engage in physical activities.

- *Pranamaya kosha tamas imbalance:* Tamas can lead to blocked or stagnant energy in the body. An individual may feel "stuck" or unable to generate the vital life force energy (prana) necessary for overall well-being.

- *Manomaya kosha tamas imbalance:* The mental sheath is profoundly affected by tamas. An imbalance in tamas can lead to mental fog, confusion, and a lack of clarity. Individuals may find it difficult to concentrate, make decisions, or engage in productive thinking.

- *Vijnanamaya kosha tamas imbalance:* Tamas can inhibit access to higher wisdom and inner guidance. An individual may struggle to connect with their inner wisdom and intuition, leading to a sense of spiritual stagnation.

- *Anandamaya kosha tamas imbalance:* Tamas can obstruct the experience of inner joy and bliss. An individual may feel emotionally numb, disconnected from their inner source of happiness, and may seek external substances or distractions to fill the void.

Social determinants of health

Factors such as socio-economic status, education, physical environment, employment, and social support networks can influence nutritional status, exposure to toxins, physical activity levels, and access to healthcare. By assessing these social determinants of health we can gain a comprehensive view of the external factors influencing the health of all of the koshas, especially the annamaya kosha.

SOCIAL DETERMINANTS OF HEALTH SCREENING SURVEY

In this section, you are asked to share your social determinants of health (SDOH). These are different areas of your life that have an impact on your health. For each category, give a rating from 1 to 5. A rating of 1 means there might be some challenges in that area, while 5 means things are going great. Having an understanding of these SDOH will help us tailor your yoga program to best suit your needs.

Economic stability

☐ Unemployed, no source of income [1 point]
☐ Below poverty line [2 points]
☐ Near poverty line [3 points]
☐ Middle income [4 points]
☐ High income, financially stable [5 points]

Education access

☐ No access to education [1 point]
☐ Limited access (e.g., only primary school) [2 points]
☐ Secondary school completed [3 points]
☐ Some college or vocational training [4 points]
☐ College degree or higher [5 points]

Social and community engagement

☐ Isolated, no community support [1 point]
☐ Rare community involvement or support [2 points]
☐ Moderate community support [3 points]
☐ Active in community, but limited support [4 points]
☐ Strong community ties and robust support [5 points]

Access to healthcare

☐ No access to healthcare [1 point]
☐ Limited access (e.g. only emergency services) [2 points]
☐ Regular primary care, but no specialists [3 points]
☐ Access to primary care and some specialists [4 points]
☐ Comprehensive healthcare access [5 points]

Housing and neighborhood

☐ Homeless or unstable housing [1 point]
☐ Stable housing but in an unsafe neighborhood [2 points]
☐ Safe neighborhood, but limited amenities [3 points]
☐ Safe neighborhood with some amenities [4 points]
☐ Safe neighborhood with ample amenities and recreational spaces [5 points]

Healthy food access

☐ No access to healthy foods, reliant on processed foods [1 point]
☐ Limited access to healthy foods [2 points]
☐ Occasional access to healthy foods [3 points]
☐ Regular access to healthy foods but with some reliance on processed options [4 points]
☐ Consistent access to diverse, healthy food choices [5 points]

Cultural and social engagement

☐ No engagement in societal activities [1 point]
☐ Rare participation [2 points]
☐ Occasional participation in societal activities [3 points]
☐ Regular participation, but not leading roles [4 points]
☐ Active leadership or regular involvement in societal activities [5 points]

Employment and working conditions

☐ Not employed at this time [1 point]
☐ Non-dependable work or working conditions [2 points]
☐ Employment in a toxic or unsafe environment [3 points]
☐ Supportive and safe work environment [4 points]
☐ Thriving and secure work environment [5 points]

Scoring for social determinants of health

Total points: . . . . /45

Social determinants of health inclusivity recommendations

- **35–45 points:** Minimal priority for services. The client seems to be well supported in most areas. They might not require immediate service referrals, but can be provided with resources for future reference.

- **24–34 points:** Low priority for services. The client has minimal challenges. They might benefit from a few specific services.

- **13–23 points:** Moderate priority for services. The client has moderate challenges in some areas. Referrals and assistance in specific areas are recommended.

- **8–12 points:** High priority for services. The client has significant challenges in multiple areas. Immediate referrals and assistance are recommended.

Although we are unable to change our client's social determinants of health, we can meet them where they are by acknowledging that the social determinants of health are a key part of our client's lived experience, and therefore they play a key role in evidence-informed practice. The following are some ways we can practice sensitivity to the social determinants of health when co-creating a one-on-one yoga program.

ECONOMIC STABILITY

- *Referrals:* If the client scored 1 or 2, consider referring to employment agencies, vocational training, or financial literacy programs.

- *Affordability:* Offer sliding scale fees, donation-based classes, or scholarships to make yoga more accessible.

- *Employment:* Consider scheduling flexibility with classes available at different times of the day or on weekends to cater to varying work schedules.

EDUCATION ACCESS

- *Referrals:* If the client scored 1 or 2, consider referring to adult education programs, scholarship opportunities, or vocational training.

- *Tailored instruction:* Recognize varying educational backgrounds, and ensure instructions are clear and concise, avoiding jargon.

- *Resources:* Provide handouts, online resources, or videos to reinforce practice at home.

SOCIAL AND COMMUNITY CONTEXT

- *Referrals:* If the client scored 1 or 2, consider recommending community engagement activities, support groups, or social clubs.

- *Community building:* Facilitate group classes or workshops that foster social connections and support.

- *Cultural competence:* Respect and acknowledge diverse backgrounds, integrating practices or teachings that resonate with various cultural groups.

ACCESS TO HEALTHCARE

- *Referrals:* If the client scored 1 or 2, refer to local healthcare providers, clinics, or mental health services.

- *Specialized training:* Instructors should be trained to work with individuals with specific health challenges or conditions.

- *Collaboration with healthcare providers:* Develop partnerships with local health organizations for referrals and co-designed interventions.

NEIGHBORHOOD AND BUILT ENVIRONMENT

- *Referrals:* If the client scored 1 or 2, consider referring to housing assistance programs, community safety initiatives, or local recreational activities.

- *Accessibility:* Choose venues that are easily accessible by public transport and ensure the facility is disability-friendly.

- *Outdoor sessions:* Organize sessions in local parks or green spaces to make use of natural surroundings for a more rejuvenating practice.

HEALTHY FOOD ACCESS

- *Referrals:* If the client scored 1 or 2, consider referring to local food banks, nutrition classes, or community gardens.

- *Nutrition workshops:* Integrate workshops on mindful eating or basic nutrition principles as a part of the yoga program.

- *Community gardens:* Collaborate with local community gardens to offer sessions that combine yoga with gardening, emphasizing the connection between nourishment, movement, and well-being.

CULTURAL AND SOCIAL ENGAGEMENT

- *Referrals:* If the client scored 1 or 2, recommend local community events, workshops, or volunteer opportunities.

- *Outreach programs:* Offer classes in community centers, schools, or elder care facilities.

- *Volunteer opportunities:* Encourage students to engage in community service or offer karma yoga opportunities where they can give back.

These recommendations are general in nature and can be tailored to your client's individual needs and circumstances. It might also be beneficial to collaborate with local service providers to ensure the most accurate and helpful referrals.

Lifestyle medicine—daily habits

The physical body's health is a direct result of daily habits and lifestyle choices. By understanding and addressing lifestyle factors, the well-being of the annamaya kosha can be enhanced, preventing diseases and promoting overall health. Lifestyle medicine focuses on the use of a whole food, plant-predominant dietary lifestyle, regular physical activity, restorative sleep, stress management, avoidance of risky substances, and positive social connection as primary therapeutic modalities.

LIFESTYLE MEDICINE SCREENING SURVEY

In this yoga lifestyle assessment, our aim is to gain a holistic understanding of your present-day lifestyle habits. The details you share will enable us to provide personalized yoga practices and guidance that harmonize with your individual circumstances. While completing this assessment, please reflect on each question and select responses that genuinely mirror your current lifestyle and feelings. Keep in mind this process is all about illuminating your current path in yoga, helping to steer your future steps.

Diet and nutrition
How many servings of fruits and vegetables do you consume daily?

- ☐ 0–1 [0 points]
- ☐ 2–3 [1 point]
- ☐ 4–5 [2 points]
- ☐ More than 5 [3 points]

How often do you consume processed foods (like chips, cookies, fast food)?

- ☐ Rarely or never [3 points]
- ☐ 1–2 times a week [2 point]
- ☐ 3–4 times a week [1 points]
- ☐ Daily or almost daily [0 points]

Physical activity
On average, how many minutes of moderate to vigorous physical activity do you engage in per week?

- ☐ Less than 30 minutes [1 point]
- ☐ 30–150 minutes [2 points]
- ☐ More than 150 minutes [3 points]

How often do you engage in stretching or flexibility exercises?

- ☐ Rarely or never [0 points]
- ☐ 1–2 times a week [1 point]
- ☐ 3–4 times a week [2 points]
- ☐ Daily or almost daily [3 points]

Sleep
On average, how many hours of quality sleep do you get each night?

- ☐ 5 hours or less [0 points]
- ☐ 6-7 hours [1 point]
- ☐ 7-8 hours [2 points]
- ☐ 8 or more hours [3 points]

How often do you feel rested upon waking?

- ☐ Rarely or never [0 points]
- ☐ Sometimes [1 point]
- ☐ Most of the time [2 points]
- ☐ Always [3 points]

Stress management

How would you rate your current stress level?

- ☐ Low [3 points]
- ☐ Moderate [2 point]
- ☐ High [1 points]
- ☐ Very high [0 points]

How often do you practice relaxation techniques (such as meditation, deep breathing, progressive muscle relaxation)?

- ☐ Rarely or never [0 points]
- ☐ 1–2 times a week [1 point]
- ☐ 3–4 times a week [2 points]
- ☐ Daily or almost daily [3 points]

Tobacco, alcohol, and recreational substances

Do you currently use tobacco products?

- ☐ Yes [0 points]
- ☐ No [3 points]

How often do you consume alcoholic beverages and/or recreational substances?

- ☐ Rarely or never [3 points]
- ☐ 1–2 times a week [2 points]
- ☐ 3–4 times a week [1 points]
- ☐ Daily or almost daily [0 points]

Scoring for lifestyle medicine

Total points . . . . /30 points

Lifestyle medicine inclusivity recommendations

- **23–30 points:** Minimal priority for support. This client has an excellent commitment to a health-centric lifestyle, and needs only general encouragement to continue their current path.

- **15–22 points:** Low priority for support. This client is engaging in mostly healthy habits, and may need a low degree of support to attune their lifestyle plans to align to goals.

- **7–14 points:** Moderate priority for support. This client needs support in modifying their lifestyle habits, and could benefit from a peer coach or professional coach.

- **0–6 points:** High priority for support. This client needs significant support for their overall lifestyle, and may benefit from the support of a coach trained in behavior change and motivation and/or an allied health professional.

As yoga professionals working in one-on-one settings, we have the opportunity to support our clients in making healthier choices in their lives, or "off the mat." As you review the clients' responses to their habits in the lifestyle medicine questionnaire, you can help them to explore ways that they can bring yoga into their lives—as part of their commitment to a healthier lifestyle. Here are a few ways we can support them in doing so, while keeping inclusivity and cultural sensitivity top of mind.

NUTRITION

- *Yogic principles:* Introduce the concept of a "sattvic" diet in yoga, which emphasizes pure, clean, and wholesome foods. Explain how yoga philosophy views food as energy for both the body and mind.

- *Inclusive approach:* Respect for diverse dietary practices and religious food restrictions. Encourage incorporating regional and seasonal foods. Keep in mind that some clients may live in a food desert, where fresh food is not available.

- *Cultural sensitivity:* Highlight how many traditional diets globally align with sattvic principles, making connections with various cultures.

EXERCISE

- *Yogic principles:* Importance of asanas (postures) in enhancing physical strength, flexibility, and endurance.

- *Inclusive approach:* Modifications for different abilities, ages, and body types. Introduce chair yoga, prenatal yoga, etc.

- *Cultural sensitivity:* Infusion of cultural elements in music, setting, or even style, like blending yoga with traditional dances or practices.

SLEEP

- *Yogic principles:* The role of yoga nidra (yogic sleep) and restorative yoga in improving sleep quality.

- *Inclusive approach:* Addressing varied sleep challenges, from insomnia to night shifts.

- *Cultural sensitivity:* Recognize and respect traditional sleep practices and routines from various cultures.

STRESS MANAGEMENT

- *Yogic principles:* Introduce pranayama (breathing exercises) and meditation for mental calmness and clarity.

- *Inclusive approach:* Tailor stress management techniques for different individuals, recognizing that the same technique may be calming to one client but aggravating to another. Support the client in finding their own practices for stress management, while staying sensitive to their social determinants of health.

- *Cultural sensitivity:* Incorporate diverse meditation practices like chanting, drumming, or using culturally relevant symbols and stories to explain stress relief.

SMOKING CESSATION

- *Yogic principles:* Introduce the yamas and niyamas, focusing on the concepts of ahimsa (non-harming) to oneself and saucha (purity), to inspire individuals to lead a cleaner, smoke-free life.

- *Inclusive approach:* Recognize the societal pressures and potential genetic predispositions towards smoking.

- *Cultural sensitivity:* Understand cultural rituals involving smoking, and provide alternatives or modifications to those rituals, such as share circles and chanting.

RESPONSIBLE USE OF ALCOHOL AND RECREATIONAL SUBSTANCES

- *Yogic principles:* Explore yoga's emphasis on mindfulness and conscious living, promoting self-awareness of someone's actions and their effects.

- *Inclusive approach:* Recognize the societal pressures and potential genetic predispositions towards alcohol.

- *Cultural sensitivity:* Understand cultural rituals involving alcohol, and provide alternatives or modifications to those rituals using yoga's mindfulness principles.

Pranamaya kosha screening surveys

The pranamaya kosha, often translated as the "energetic sheath" or "vital energy layer," is the kosha (sheath) that encapsulates the human experience according to yogic philosophy. It is the layer concerned with the vital life force known as prana, and encompasses the body's energetic anatomy, including the chakras (energy centers) and nadis (energy channels). Assessing the state of someone's pranamaya kosha is essential for a deeper understanding of overall health, vitality, and well-being.

Pranamaya holistic screening options

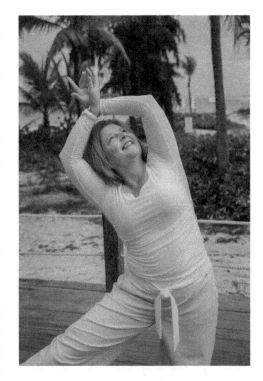

When assessing the pranamaya kosha, it's beneficial to approach the process holistically, considering various signs and feedback mechanisms. It's also helpful to consult with experienced practitioners, especially when unfamiliar with certain assessment methods. And, as always, personal experiences and insights are of paramount importance in understanding someone's energetic health.

- *Observation of breath:* The most direct way to understand the pranamaya kosha is through observing the breath. Irregularities, shallowness, or other anomalies in the breathing pattern can indicate an imbalance in the pranamaya kosha. We can ask the client to notice their breath, or we can observe their breath.

- *Energy levels:* We can ask the client what their overall energy level is on a scale of 1–10, with 10 being high. We can also ask them to use three words to describe their current energy level. A general feeling of fatigue, lethargy, or lack of vitality can indicate disturbances in the pranamaya kosha.

- *Emotional state:* We can ask the client what their overall emotional state is, on a scale of 1–10, with 10 being best. We can also ask them to use three words to describe their current emotional state. Since emotions are closely linked to pranic flow, frequent mood swings, heightened emotional reactions, or a general sense of emotional instability can hint at imbalances in this sheath.

- *Body scans and somatics:* We can ask the client to take a moment of interoception to scan their body, or move mindfully, and to tell us what they notice generally. We can also ask them to describe where they feel more or less open, more or less vibrant, more or less energetic.

- *Intuitive insights:* We can observe the client with our own intuitive capabilities, and we can ask the client to notice themselves intuitively. A favorite question here is "What do you notice within yourself?" Sometimes I also use specific question to focus their intuitive intention: "If your ___ could speak, what would it say?" Here we can say body, heart, mind, or spirit, based on what the client wants to focus on and/or what their health history has indicated we may want to focus on together. In this way, we are encouraging them to reflect on their felt state of their pranamaya kosha, and we are also reinforcing their ability to go within themselves, and to listen to their intuition. This is yoga!

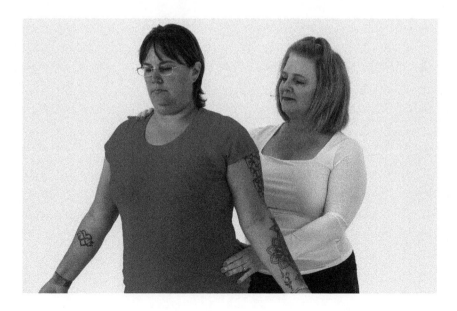

Pranamaya kosha vayu screening survey

In Ayurvedic philosophy, the vayus represent five vital winds or energies that govern specific physiological and psychological functions within our body. Each vayu plays a pivotal role in ensuring our overall well-being, from regulating our digestive system to guiding our emotional responses. By understanding and aligning with these inherent forces, we can cultivate a harmonious state of health, balance, and vitality. This assessment is designed to gauge the state of your vayus, providing insights into areas of balance and potential imbalances.

VAYU SCREENING SURVEY

1. Prana vayu (inward and upward movement—chest region)

How is your inhalation during breathing?

☐ Deep [3 points]
☐ Shallow [2 points]
☐ Irregular [1 point]

Do you often experience anxiety or fearful thoughts?

☐ Yes [1 point]
☐ No [3 points]

Any issues related to the heart or lungs:

. . . . [−1 point for each issue related to heart]

. . . . [−1 point for each issue related to lungs]

2. Apana vayu (downward and outward movement—lower abdomen)

How regular are your bowel movements?

☐ Regular [3 points]
☐ Irregular [1 point]

Frequency of urination:

☐ Normal [3 points]
☐ Frequent [2 points]
☐ Less frequent [1 point]

3. Samana vayu (centering movement—navel region)

How is your digestion?

☐ Good [3 points]
☐ Slow [2 points]
☐ Fast [1 point]

Do you often feel bloated or have gas?

☐ Yes [1 point]
☐ No [3 points]

Any food intolerances or allergies:

. . . . [−1 point for food intolerance/s]

. . . . [−1 point for allergy/ies]

4. Udana vayu (upward and outward movement—throat and head region)

Do you have clarity in speech and expression?

☐ Yes [3 points]
☐ No [1 point]

Any issues related to the thyroid or throat:

. . . . [−1 point for thyroid issue/s]

. . . . [−1 point for throat issue/s]

How is your memory and thought clarity?

☐ Good [3 points]
☐ Average [2 points]
☐ Poor [1 point]

5. Vyana vayu (circulation throughout the body)

How would you describe your overall circulation?

☐ Good [3 points]
☐ Average [2 points]
☐ Poor [1 point]

Do you often feel fatigued or lethargic?

☐ Yes [1 point]
☐ No [3 points]

Any issues with joint mobility or muscle flexibility?

. . . . [−1 point for joint mobility issue/s]

. . . . [−1 point for muscle flexibility issue/s]

Scoring for vayus

Total prana vayu: . . . ./6

Total apana vayu: . . . ./6

Total samana vayu: . . . . /6

Total udana vayu: . . . ./6

Total vyana vayu: . . . ./6

Total vayus: . . . ./30

Vayu inclusivity recommendations

A balanced vayu system ensures optimal health and well-being. If any imbalances are detected, consider seeking guidance from an Ayurvedic practitioner or adopting relevant practices to bring harmony to the specific vayu.

- For the vayus overall, calculate the total points of all vayus:

- **20–30 points:** High-level vitality; aim to continue to manage vayus optimally.

- **10–20 points:** Medium-level vitality; aim to increase vitality in deficient areas.

- **<9 points:** Low vitality and high burnout risk; support client in improving energy and consider referring client as needed for energy balance.

Part 2: Vitality type screening (individual vayus)

- For each vayu category, calculate the total points:

- **5–6 points:** This vayu is balanced and functioning optimally.

- **3–4 points:** This vayu is slightly imbalanced and may need attention.

- **<2 points:** This vayu is significantly imbalanced and requires immediate attention and practices to restore balance.

Pranamaya kosha chakra screening survey

The chakras, ancient Sanskrit for wheel, represent the seven primary energy centers in the body. Each chakra regulates different aspects of our physical, emotional, mental, and spiritual well-being. When balanced, they promote harmony, vitality, and alignment. However, life's various challenges and experiences can lead to imbalances in these energy centers, manifesting in various ways, from emotional discomfort to physical ailments.

CHAKRA BALANCE SCREENING SURVEY: EXPLORING YOUR ENERGETIC BODY

This chakra assessment offers you a unique lens to introspect and gauge the alignment and balance of your chakras. By responding genuinely to each statement, you will get a glimpse into which of your chakras are flourishing, and which might be seeking your attention.

For each statement, rate how often you resonate with it on a scale of 1 to 5, with 1 being "Rarely" and 5 being "Always."

Root chakra (muladhara)

. . . . /5: I feel grounded and connected to the earth.

. . . . /5: I have a strong sense of security and stability in my life.

Sacral chakra (svadhisthana)

. . . . /5: I feel in touch with my emotions and can express them.

. . . . /5: I enjoy physical sensations and experiences.

Solar plexus chakra (manipura)

. . . . /5: I feel confident in my decisions.

. . . . /5: I have a strong sense of personal power and motivation.

Heart chakra (anahata)

. . . . /5: I can give and receive love easily.

. . . . /5: I feel a deep sense of inner peace and compassion.

Throat chakra (vishuddha)

. . . . /5: I am comfortable speaking my truth and expressing myself.

. . . . /5: I feel heard and understood by others.

Third eye chakra (ajna)

. . . . /5: I have strong intuition and often trust my inner guidance.

. . . . /5: I can visualize with clarity and have vivid dreams.

Crown chakra (sahasrara)

. . . . /5: I feel a deep connection to a higher power or the universe.

. . . . /5: Moments of enlightenment or profound understanding come to me naturally.

Scoring for chakras

Total points: . . . . /70

Chakra inclusivity recommendations

Understanding your dominant chakras and those that may need attention can guide you towards practices and meditations that enhance your overall energetic health. Consider consulting with a holistic healer or meditation expert to dive deeper into any imbalances detected.

PART 1: OVERALL EMOTIONAL ENERGY ASSESSMENT (ALL CHAKRAS)

- For the chakras overall, calculate the total points of all seven of the chakras:

- **57–70 points:** Highly aligned and balanced.

- **43–56 points:** Moderately aligned, minor imbalances.

- **29–42 points:** Somewhat misaligned, consider practices to restore balance.

- **14–28 points:** Misaligned and requires attention and a program to work towards rebalance. A referral may be needed.

PART 2: EMOTIONAL ENERGY ASSESSMENT BY TYPE (INDIVIDUAL CHAKRAS)

- For each chakra category, calculate the total points:

- **7–10 points:** This chakra is balanced and functioning optimally.

- **4–6 points:** This chakra is slightly imbalanced and may need attention.

- **<4 points:** This chakra is significantly imbalanced and requires immediate attention and practices to restore balance.

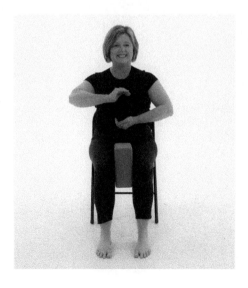

MANOMAYA KOSHA SCREENING SURVEY: SELF-AWARENESS, THOUGHTS, FEELINGS, AND SENSES

The manomaya kosha, or the "mental sheath," plays a significant role in how we perceive, think, feel, and relate with the world around us. It encompasses our thoughts, emotions, beliefs, perceptions, and more. Delving into an understanding of this layer can offer profound insights into our mental well-being and patterns of thinking and feeling. This assessment is designed to provide a snapshot of your manomaya kosha. By responding to each question you'll be better positioned to recognize patterns, areas of strength, and potential areas for growth.

Self-awareness

I feel connected to my inner self during challenging times:

- ☐ Never [0 points]
- ☐ Rarely [1 point]
- ☐ Sometimes [2 points]
- ☐ Often [3 points]
- ☐ Always [4 points]

I utilize yoga or introspective practices to navigate my mental well-being:

- ☐ Never [0 points]
- ☐ Rarely [1 point]
- ☐ Sometimes [2 points]
- ☐ Often [3 points]
- ☐ Always [4 points]

Thoughts

My mind frequently races with thoughts:

- ☐ Never [4 points]
- ☐ Rarely [3 points]
- ☐ Sometimes [2 points]
- ☐ Often [1 point]
- ☐ Always [0 points]

I find it challenging to detach from negative or recurring thoughts:

- ☐ Never [4 points]
- ☐ Rarely [3 points]
- ☐ Sometimes [2 points]
- ☐ Often [1 point]
- ☐ Always [0 points]

I practice meditation or mindfulness to center my thoughts:

- ☐ Never [0 points]
- ☐ Rarely [1 point]
- ☐ Sometimes [2 points]
- ☐ Often [3 points]
- ☐ Always [4 points]

I am as kind to myself in my self-talk as I would be when talking with a dear friend:

- ☐ Never [0 points]
- ☐ Rarely [1 point]
- ☐ Sometimes [2 points]
- ☐ Often [3 points]
- ☐ Always [4 points]

Feelings

I feel overwhelmed by my emotions:

- ☐ Never [4 points]
- ☐ Rarely [3 points]
- ☐ Sometimes [2 points]
- ☐ Often [1 point]
- ☐ Always [0 points]

I find it hard to think or move forward without overthinking:

- ☐ Never [4 points]
- ☐ Rarely [3 points]
- ☐ Sometimes [2 points]
- ☐ Often [1 point]
- ☐ Always [0 points]

I seek to suppress or avoid my feelings rather than face them:

☐ Never [4 points]
☐ Rarely [3 points]
☐ Sometimes [2 points]
☐ Often [1 point]
☐ Always [0 points]

I often reflect on my emotions to understand their origin:

☐ Never [0 points]
☐ Rarely [1 point]
☐ Sometimes [2 points]
☐ Often [3 points]
☐ Always [4 points]

Scoring for Manomya kosha

Total points: .... /40

Manomaya kosha inclusivity recommendations

- **31–40 points:** High self-awareness and emotional balance. Empower the client to continue their self-awareness and emotional balance efforts and to consider finding ways to share these skills with others (personally or professionally).

- **21–30 points:** Moderate self-awareness and emotional balance. Encourage the client to continue efforts to develop self-awareness and emotional balance; this can be part of their one-on-one yoga program.

- **11–20 points:** Developing self-awareness and emotional balance. Consider referring the client to services that support emotional and mental health.

Vijnanamaya kosha screening survey

In the journey of self-awareness and personal growth, understanding our inner realm of intellect, wisdom, and intuition is crucial. The vijnanamaya kosha, often referred to as the "wisdom body," is a layer of our being that governs these very aspects.

VIJNANAMAYA KOSHA SCREENING SURVEY

This assessment is designed to offer insights into how you navigate your inner world, from your logical reasoning and ethical understanding to your intuitive insights and subconscious connections. Reflect on your tendencies and capacities regarding decision-making, intuition, and critical thinking. Please rate each statement on a scale of 1–5, where 1 represents "Strongly disagree" and 5 represents "Strongly agree." As you progress through the survey, be honest with your responses. Remember—this isn't about achieving a "perfect score," but rather about gaining insights and understanding into your wisdom body.

Intuition and insight

. . . . /5: I often rely on my intuition to guide my decisions.

. . . . /5: I regularly have moments of deep insight or understanding about myself and the world.

. . . . /5: I can easily distinguish between my intuition and my emotional impulses.

Discernment and wisdom

. . . . /5: I can differentiate between the permanent (the self or soul) and the impermanent (physical world).

. . . . /5: I actively seek wisdom from both external sources and my inner self.

. . . . /5: I often reflect on my experiences to draw deeper meaning and understanding.

Intellectual pursuits and knowledge

. . . . /5: I engage in regular intellectual activities that challenge and grow my understanding of the self and the world.

. . . . /5: I recognize that knowledge is infinite, and I'm always eager to learn more.

. . . . /5: I can detach from my biases and beliefs to perceive situations more objectively.

Connection to the Higher Self

. . . . /5: I often feel a connection to a higher sense of Self beyond my mind and emotions.

. . . . /5: I prioritize practices that help me connect to my true nature, such as meditation or self-inquiry.

. . . . /5: I have moments where I feel a sense of unity with everything around me.

Scoring for Vijnanamaya kosha

Total points: . . . . /60

Vijnanamaya kosha inclusivity recommendations

- **45–60 points:** Moderate to high vitality in the vijnanamaya layer. The client has a strong level of spiritual well-being, showing strength in intuition, wisdom, intellectual pursuits, and connection to the Higher Self. Healthcare referrals may not be necessary unless specific issues are identified during the assessment.

- **29–44 points:** Developing vitality in the vijnanamaya layer. The client is making progress in their spiritual well-being, but may still benefit from guidance and resources to further develop their intuition, wisdom, intellectual pursuits, and connection to the Higher Self.

- **12–28 points:** Low vitality in the vijnanamaya layer. The client may benefit from referrals to explore practices and resources that can enhance their intuition, wisdom, intellectual pursuits, and connection to the Higher Self.

Anandamaya kosha screening survey

The deepest layer of our being, the anandamaya kosha, is often referred to as the "bliss sheath." It is the subtlest layer, where innate joy, contentment, and a sense of oneness with the universe reside. It is this realm where we touch the purest sense of joy, contentment, and a state of inherent happiness that is unconnected to the external circumstances of life. This sheath is not about momentary pleasures or temporary highs, but rather a sustained, profound sense of peace and well-being that resides within us.

ANANDAMAYA KOSHA SCREENING SURVEY

This survey aims to measure your connection and awareness to the anandamaya kosha by gauging your experiences and feelings related to inner joy, the sense of oneness, detachment from external desires, and the True Self's awareness. By understanding where you resonate with the statements, you'll gain insights into the areas where your connection to the anandamaya kosha is strong, and where there might be opportunities for deeper exploration and growth.

Please rate each statement on a scale of 1–5, where 1 represents "Strongly disagree" and 5 represents "Strongly agree." As you navigate the survey, approach each statement with openness and authenticity.

Connection to inner joy

. . . . /5: I often experience moments of profound joy and contentment without external reasons.

. . . . /5: I can easily tap into feelings of bliss during meditation or introspective practices.

. . . . /5: I feel a deep sense of peace and wholeness within myself.

Experience of transcendence

. . . . /5: I have had experiences where I felt connected to something greater than myself.

. . . . /5: In moments of deep meditation or reflection, I feel a sense of oneness with everything.

. . . . /5: I occasionally lose track of time and self during moments of intense joy or absorption.

Detachment from external desires

. . . . /5: I find happiness within myself rather than external achievements or possessions.

. . . . /5: My sense of contentment is not easily shaken by external challenges or disappointments.

. . . . /5: I understand that true happiness comes from within and is not dependent on external conditions.

Awareness of the True Self

.... /5: I feel a deeper sense of Self that is beyond my thoughts, emotions, and physical body.

.... /5: I recognize that my true nature is blissful and unchanging.

.... /5: My moments of deepest joy and contentment come from connecting with this inner Self.

Scoring for Anandamaya kosha

Total points:......./60

Anandamaya kosha inclusivity recommendations

- **45–60 points:** Moderate to high vitality in the anandamaya kosha. The client has a good to high level of spiritual well-being, showing strength in their connection to inner joy, experience of transcendence, detachment from external desires, and awareness of the True Self. Healthcare referrals may not be necessary unless specific issues are identified during the assessment.

- **29–44 points:** Developing vitality in the anandamaya kosha. The client is making progress in their spiritual well-being, but may still benefit from guidance and resources to further develop their connection to inner joy, experience of transcendence, detachment from external desires, and awareness of the True Self.

- **12–28 points:** Low vitality in the anandamaya kosha. The client may benefit from referrals to explore practices and resources that can enhance their connection to inner joy, experience of transcendence, detachment from external desires, and awareness of the True Self.

Summary of integrative health intake forms

As you can see, there are many dimensions of integrative health we can assess through the client's intake forms. As you consider which forms make the most sense to you and your clients, please keep in mind that we want to balance our need to learn about the client's needs with their experience of completing the forms. Since the intake form completion is technically their first engagement with us, it's important to consider ways to make the form completion process more user-friendly, such as putting the forms in an online tool and/or streamlining the forms based on the information you feel is most relevant and realistic for accurate and timely completion.

▓ STEP 3: THE CLIENT INTERVIEW

After the client has completed their consent and waiver forms (Step 1), and their integrative health intake forms (Step 2), it is time to sit down with them and to discuss what we know so far. I call this step the "client interview," and consider it as a very important segue between the intake form completion process and their asana assessment (which we will cover as Step 4 of the SOAP process). Through the interview, we have our first golden opportunity to engage live with the client as part of the co-creation of their one-on-one yoga program.

The interview session is a delicate dance of understanding, empathy, and connection, as it sets the tone for the transformative journey that lies ahead. By embracing the principles of sense-making, the wisdom of the koshas, and a coaching mindset, we can ensure that both the yoga professional (you) and the client are aligned in purpose and vision for the co-creation journey.

The power of sense-making

The sense-making framework, shown in Figure 6, was developed by Dr. Brenda Dervin[19] as part of her work in the library sciences. It was originally designed to explain the phenomenon of an individual trying to "make sense of" information they collect during the research and writing processes. However, when I was introduced to the theory in 2013, I realized that it could be applied in one-on-one yoga work with clients. Essentially I extrapolated the concepts of the theory, and applied them to our life story and our lived experience. Through my mixed-methods research, I proposed that well-being is a sense-making process—one in which an individual makes sense of their health outcomes, lived experiences, and life situations. In other words, we don't have to have a perfect life or perfect health outcomes to have well-being; instead, we can make sense of our life story in a way that generates well-being through sense-making and social support.[20]

As we examine the sense-making model from the perspective of an individual's well-being, we can see that every human is either in a state of feeling as though their life is making sense (sense-making) or feeling stuck because they don't know where they are going or how they will get there (sense-unmaking). Every individual is constantly trying to make sense of their life's narrative, drawing from their past experiences, current situations (i.e., life story plot twists), and future aspirations. The sense-making model (picture) helps us to envision how we engage in this sense-making process, and how we can envision times when life isn't making sense (i.e., sense-unmaking).

The sense-making process occurs when we know where we are (situation), where we are taking our life story next (flags), and how we will get there (bridge). It is important to note that this sense-making process depends on a sturdy bridge of beliefs, attitudes, and values—that can take us from where we are (situation) to where we want to go (flag). The sense-making process also depends on our taking an umbrella with us—which is symbolic of the cultures that are there to support us and protect us along the way from the unexpected events (e.g., rain) that can come up as we move towards where we want to take our life next.

The sense-unmaking process occurs when we don't know where we are going (i.e., we don't have a flag to head towards); we don't know how we will get there (i.e., we don't have a bridge of beliefs that will take us where we are to where we want to go); and/or we forgot we can take an umbrella to support and protect us (i.e., we don't lean on the social support and communities that can help us).

In our one-on-one yoga program interview, we can use this sense-making framework to understand how the client is, and isn't, making sense of their life story. This insight can then inform whether or not we give the client a referral and/or invite them to engage with us in a one-on-one yoga program.

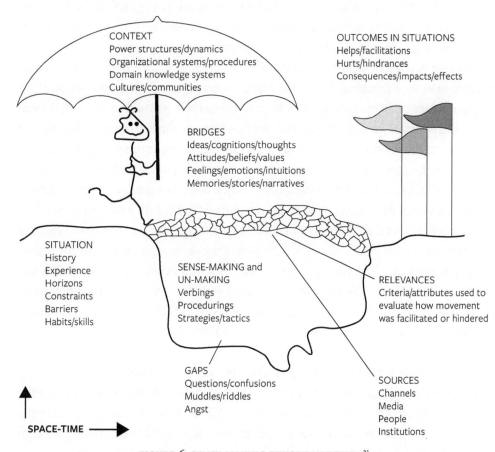

FIGURE 6: SENSE-MAKING THEORY BY DERVIN[21]

The sense-making picture offers us a "big picture" to where we are, and aren't, making sense in our lives. Using the metaphor of this framework (which is considered both a theory and a model), we are all the human on the left of the picture, at once centered and decentered (as depicted in the face that is both straight and squiggly). We are all coming from somewhere (the situation of our past) and moving towards the outcomes of the sense we are making—what we believe to be true in our life story. We may feel as though we are moving towards our goals, on the bridge of our beliefs, values, thoughts, and actions; in this way we are making sense of our life story. Or we may feel as though we don't know where we should go and/or where we should turn. In this place, we are in sense-unmaking, and we have fallen into the gap between where we are (situation) and where we want to be (flags). Here, we can't see whether we need a new bridge of beliefs, a new flag placement, or a new pathway to the flag we were aiming for. As we reflect on where we want to go next, and how we want to get there, the picture re-emerges and suddenly we are making sense again. We know where we are and where we are going and how we will get there. We also feel supported by the cultures and communities who are there for us, protecting us like the umbrella depicted in the human's hand.

I invite you to consider that every client you talk to will be in a space of sense-making or sense-unmaking. By visualizing the picture (theory), you can ask questions and stimulate dialogue to help the client to fill in their picture, or reset it, if need be. It is important to note, however, that this process must be inquiry-based, and driven by the individual. It is of vital importance that we, as the yoga professional, don't grab the pen and fill in the client's sense-making picture; it is up to the client to determine where they have been (situation); where they are (on or off the bridge of beliefs, attitudes, and values that feel supportive); where they are going (the flags of their goals); and if they are supported in the risks that will come with the journey (by carrying an umbrella). They hold the pen of the sense-making picture—because it is their sense-making process. If we were to tell the client how to write in any or all of these sense-making components, we would be taking their agency away, demotivating them, and promoting transference. It is their life to live, not ours; it is therefore their life story to make sense of and tell, and not ours.

An example of a client interview based on sense-making

Here is an example of how you can apply Dervin's sense-making model during the one-on-one yoga program interview process. Please note that this is an example and is not meant to be shared as a script; you are encouraged to co-create your own conversation with your client based on their unique sense-making picture.

1. SITUATION OR GAP: WHERE ARE WE NOW?

Before diving into the interview, acknowledge the current situation. What has led the client to seek a personal yoga program? From the sense-making perspective, this is how the client is making sense of, and finding meaning in, their current situation (and is not solely about the data they submitted in their intake form). For instance, a client may be going through significant stressors at work. However, one client may make sense of the story of this stress in a positive framing, believing that the hard work will bring the team together and produce better results. Another client may be going through the same work stress situation, but they may be not able to make sense of that stress because they see "no end in sight" for their work stress.

Interview example:

Yoga professional: "Hello [client's name]. Thank you for choosing to embark on this personal yoga journey with me. Our goal today is for me to better understand your aspirations, challenges, and preferences related to yoga, so we can co-create a program that supports you well. Do you have any questions before we begin?"
[Client asks questions and yoga professional answers them as needed.]
Yoga professional: "To start, can you share what circumstances in your health or your life led you to explore a one-on-one yoga program?"
Client: "I went through a lot of stress in my job last year, and I am told by my doctor I have to reduce stress. I realize now I can't do it alone. I want to learn more about how I can manage the stress of my job and my life because I really like my job and the people I work with. I don't want to let them down, but I don't want to let myself down either."
Yoga professional: "Thank you for sharing that. It's essential for me to understand where you're coming from so we can shape your yoga journey accordingly. I hear you saying that you have a stressful job and that you enjoy it, so you want to learn how to cope with that work stress through your yoga program. Do I have that right?"

Notice in this reflection that the yoga professional is staying neutral in their response, and staying focused on where the client is in their sense-making picture. In this case, it is the client's conflict between loving a job that is stressful, liking her colleagues, and realizing she needs to prioritize her health and stress management so she can keep enjoying her life and her work. Because she is in conflict, she is in the gap. This means that she isn't sure which flag to choose (i.e., staying in a job because she likes her colleagues or leaving a profession because it is stressful).

2. FLAGS (OUTCOME GOALS): WHERE ARE WE GOING?
The flags in Dervin's sense-making model are symbolic of the goals, or milestones, we want to achieve. In the case of a one-on-one yoga client interview, we can encourage the client to tell us more about the vision they would like to achieve through the program. In this way we keep our focus on the future, while bringing hope and potentiality into the conversation. This is a shift in the conversation out of the conflict of the client's current situation or gap, and all of the discomfort that comes

with it, into the possibilities of what it would be like without this conflict (or with it resolved).

Interview example:

Yoga professional: "Given your focus on work stress management, what do you hope to achieve through this yoga program?"

Client: "I want to stop feeling torn between my work and my health and my life. There just aren't enough hours in the day, and I feel as though no one is getting the best of me—including me."

Yoga professional: "I am glad to hear that you want to stop feeling torn. Can you tell me what that looks like for you—that place of feeling that your work, your life, and your health are all feeling like they are getting the best of you?"

Notice that the client tried to pull the conversation backwards, into her discomfort. We can skillfully ask questions focused on the future, to shift our attention into the sense-making process—to start to "fill in the sense-making picture." As the client starts to narrate the future state, or flags (vision), the yoga professional can ask additional questions to fill in this picture of what the client's new world will look like—when they realize their vision. Much like we want to visualize a vacation before we go through the work to pack and travel, it's important that the client has this vision (flags) in mind as part of the sense-making process.

3. GAP OF SENSE-UNMAKING: NOT KNOWING WHERE
WE ARE OR WHERE WE ARE GOING

When we look closely at Dervin's model (theory of sense-making), we can see that the gap is a specific experience of sense-unmaking. Here we feel as though we have lost ourselves somewhere on our journey. The gap is a place where the client is not quite sure where they are and/or where they are going. There are many reasons that gaps can occur for clients. For example, the client may find themselves not knowing where they want to go next. It is as though they are stuck on the road trying to decide where they should head next. Or they may find themself taking a detour off their bridge. (We'll learn more about the bridge of beliefs in a moment; suffice to say that this experience of the gap feels like we don't know if what we thought was true really is true. This can be a positive experience (e.g. releasing a limiting belief), or not (e.g. feeling let down by someone you care for).

However they find themselves in a gap, the client who is here feels as though they are lost, alone, and in the dark, "not knowing which way to turn or where to go next." It can also feel like the dark night of the soul. Notice that these phrases we use every day to explain times of frustration or difficulty have an imagery in them—an imagery that correlates with the sense-making picture and Dervin's description of the gap as a place of angst and confusion.

The key to supporting the client's sense-making process (through the practice of co-creation) is to encourage them to orient to their current situation, and to where they are going (flags). Essentially, we repeat steps 1 and 2 until the client can start to see their sense-making picture emerge.

If a client is having trouble seeing their vision of success, you might encourage them to draw a picture or complete a vision board. If they still have difficulty looking forward into the future, this may be time to refer the client to mental health support. This referral must be handled carefully because we are not diagnosing or prescribing the client, to stay in our scope of practice. At the same time, our scope as yoga professionals is to focus on where the client is, and where they are going. If they can't focus their attention on moving forward, and are too caught up in looking back at the past or down into the present (without the ability to look up and out into the future), then I would encourage them to seek professional mental health support for that process.

4. BRIDGE OF BELIEFS: SENSE-MAKING AS MOVING FORWARD AND WELL-BEING (VERB)

When the client gets back to an awareness of their situation and their flags (and is no longer in the gap), the sense-making process begins again. Here the client may be able to link where they are now to where they want to go—through the bridge of their beliefs.

In our scenario, the client has started out stuck in her situation, believing that her goals for her health, her work, and her life are all taking her in different directions. She is immobilized by knowing that no matter which way she goes, she will find herself ignoring the other two flags. This is why she has sought our help, through the one-on-one yoga program.

Here we can help the client by supporting her in the realization that her desired flags don't need to be thought of as three different directions in her life story; instead, they can be considered as co-located. In this way, we can help the client rethink her efforts towards self-care and health as not disparate or distracting for her work and life goals; instead, she can begin reconceptualizing that her work will be enhanced even as she invests time and energy into her health. As she buys into this possibility, she is essentially building a new bridge of belief: she is thinking differently about her dilemma.

It is important that we don't "grab the flags" for the client by telling her what goals to make and that we don't tell her what to think (i.e., do the construction work in her thought process for her). Instead, we can support her in making this realization by herself. Here is an example of how we might do this carefully in the client interview process.

Interview example:

Yoga professional: "I'm hearing you say that you would love to see yourself in a place where your health, your work, and your life are all getting along, and feeling connected together. How could you rethink your health and your work as not an 'either/or' but as an 'and'?"

Client: "You're right that I think of them as either/or. I am not sure what you mean by the 'and.'"

Yoga professional: "How about an example. You have a work call and you want to go for a walk. How could you put these together as an 'and,' instead of deciding between them?"

Client: "Some work calls have to be online but others could be by phone. I suppose I could take one of my daily work calls on a daily walk."

Yoga professional: "How would that feel to combine a health habit with a work habit?"

Client: "It feels less hard actually—lighter even. It feels like I'm not fighting within myself."

Yoga professional: "How else could you find ways to bring your goals for health and your work demands together, so you don't feel as though you're fighting within yourself?"

5. UMBRELLA (CULTURE AND COMMUNITY FOR SOCIAL SUPPORT)

In the sense-making picture, the human is holding an umbrella, which is a metaphor for being shielded from rain and adversity. The umbrella represents the communities and cultures that support us, providing us with social support and compassion. Just as we may not always need an umbrella but it is good to know it is there if we should need it, social and community support function in much the same way. We can feel confident heading towards our goals knowing that we have a plan for adversity, and that we don't have to make the journey alone.

Interview example:

Yoga professional: "When you think about your efforts to take care of yourself this week, who can help you in keeping your commitment to your self?"

Client: "My husband has been telling me I need to stop putting everyone and everything else first. I think I could ask him to hold me accountable and to make sure I am doing the program."

Yoga professional: "That sounds like a good idea. How does that feel to ask for his support?"

Client: "It feels good because I know he will be happy that I am finally doing this. But I am also a little nervous because I have had a hard time with this in the past and I may not be able to be perfect at this."

Yoga professional: "Well, the good news is that I am here to support you too, and in yoga we don't aim for perfection. We aim for self-realization. We are here to learn what does and doesn't work for you, so everything we try is simply an experiment—something to explore. How does it feel to think of it that way?"

Notice in this discussion that the yoga professional helped the client to examine another "cobblestone" on the bridge of belief—the belief that she won't be able to succeed because she wasn't able to succeed in the past. The yoga professional helped her to replace this cobblestone with a new belief—that yoga is an accepting practice of self-realization, not perfection. In this way, the yoga professional helped her to feel more confident on the "road ahead" (aka bridge of beliefs).

Interview recap

At the end of the interview, we can use sense-making to review with the client where they are in their priorities, and where they want to go for their vision. We can also help them to imagine and visualize the picture of sense-making—which helps them to see beyond the gaps they may find themselves in. Here's an example from our scenario.

Yoga professional: "So let's recap what we discovered today. We know that you have been feeling like you are constantly having to choose between your work, your life, and your health—and that you are ready to reduce stress. We also know that we are going to build your program that helps you to get to your vision—a place where your life, your work, and your health are all getting along. We'll build the program together, to explore what strategies do and don't work for you. For example, this week, we'll see if the walking work call is something you want to include in your program, or if we need to brainstorm another option. Together we are going to build a plan that has you feeling like you are moving forward, instead of feeling pulled in too many directions. And you are going to ask your husband for support in staying accountable to the plan, beyond the work we will do together. Would you agree with this recap, or would you revise it?"

Notice that we are giving the client the opportunity to hear through our words the painting of the sense-making picture. In this narrative, the yoga professional illuminated the situation, the gap, the flags, and the new beliefs on the bridge. They also asked the client to review the recap, to make sure that the client has the ultimate ownership of the "pen" of writing their life story. In the act of asking the client to confirm whether or not the recap is accurate, we are ensuring that we are staying person-centered. Another strategy is to ask the client to do the recap, and for the yoga professional to adjust it as needed. Either way, the emphasis is on ensuring that the client is in charge of their sense-making picture, and their life story.

STEP 4: ASANA ASSESSMENT SESSION

After gathering so much information in Steps 1 through 3, it may be hard to believe we have more information to gather! However, if we are going to co-create a yoga program that includes asanas, it's important that we also include an asana assessment session in our five-step SOAP process. In this section, we'll explore how we can prepare for and conduct an asana-based assessment session (rather than a biomechanic movement-based one).

I have found in my private practice and in my work training yoga instructors and yoga therapists that using asanas (rather than biomechanic movement protocols) for the client's physical assessment offers two benefits. First, the client is automatically introduced to yoga postures in this process. In this way, they are learning the names of postures and details about how to perform them safely, which is especially important for clients who are new to yoga who also have medical concerns. Second, the client also has the opportunity to experience some of the general experience of a full one-on-one yoga session—to preview what this will be like. This preview of our future work goes a long way to building trust with the client, as well as their buy-in.

Preparing for the asana assessment
Part 1: Know the rules of the asana assessment road

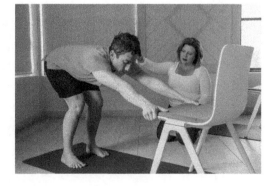

If you are licensed to drive a car, you know that it's important that you know the rules of the road before you begin your journey. In a similar way, I have developed these rules for the asana assessment road, to support both you and your client in promoting a safe and healthy drive—in this case, an asana assessment session. These rules of the road are also recommended for yoga sessions, as long as they are in keeping with your own scope of practice and the client's medical guidance and intuitive knowledge.

- *Move in and out of neutral spine:* There is an old saying that there is a little mountain in every pose. In the same way, we can move in and out of yoga postures through a neutral spine. A neutral spine offers the perfect balance between flexibility and strength. Encourage clients to:

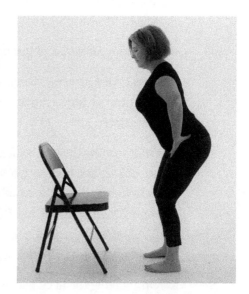

  - Bend their knees and/or elbows to find and maintain this neutral position

  - Ensure transitions in and out of poses are anchored in this neutral position for core stability

  - Avoid simultaneous complex spinal movements, thereby emphasizing simplicity

  - Follow the "fold like a folder" technique, so that they can move from the center

  - Transition in and out of postures from a neutral spine to avoid undue risk.

- *Open with love (from the heart center, not the lumbar spine):* The heart center is not just a physical region; it also represents love, openness, and compassion, which is integral to our yoga heritage and philosophy. To harness this energy:

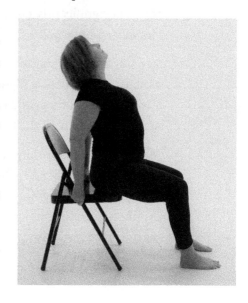

  - Focus on keeping the spine elongated and smooth, devoid of abrupt transitions

  - Target the thoracic spine when

emphasizing openness, steering clear of the cervical and lumbar regions, which can be more injury-prone

- Recognize the flow from elongation to extension, and from restful elongation to flexion, ensuring a balanced and harmonious movement sequence

- Keep the cervical and lumbar sections of the spine neutral.

- *Keep the neck neutral:* Neck safety is of the utmost importance. To ensure client safety:

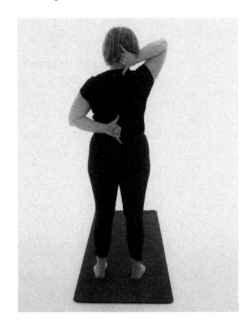

  - Omit turning the head when the hips are positioned higher than the head, as in the case of Adho Mukha Svanasana (Downward Facing Dog), Setu Bandha Sarvangasana (Bridge Pose), and any type of shoulder stand

  - Omit taking the neck backward (cervical spine compression)

  - Use caution when turning the head from the neck—moving slowly with awareness.

- *Microbend to befriend:*

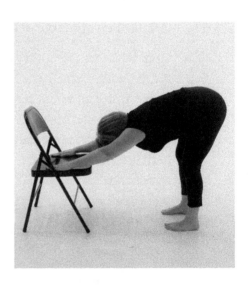

  - Microbending is a nuanced technique that can significantly enhance pose stability and safety.

  - In poses that challenge balance, such as standing postures, a slight bend in the knees can offer added stability and reduce strain on the lower back.

  - Similarly, when working with arm balances, a microbend in the elbows can assist in distributing weight evenly and preventing undue stress on the upper back.

- *Engage the core chain through the bandhas:* The ancient yogic concept of bandhas refers to the "energy locks" in our body. Engaging these locks can significantly enhance posture stability and energy flow:

  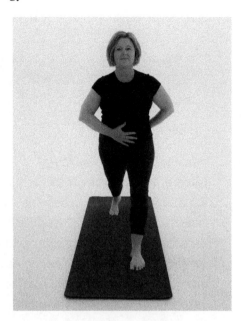

  - *Pada bandha* engages the arches of the feet, promoting stability.

  - *Mula bandha,* or the pelvic floor lift, strengthens the core and supports the spine.

  - *Udiyana bandha* engages the transversus abdominus, further fortifying the core.

  - *Jalandara bandha* ensures neck stability, particularly essential in poses that strain the cervical spine.

  - Lastly, *hasta bandha* offers support in weight-bearing poses involving the hands.

Although each client will also have their own safety concerns based on their own unique health history, these rules of the road are designed to support general safety for all clients. Through mindful integration of these principles, yoga professionals can offer sessions that are both safe as well as profoundly impactful.

Part 2: Driving the asanas safely with the traffic light method

With these safety tips in mind, it's time to get behind the wheel (metaphorically speaking) to begin driving the asana assessments. In my private yoga teacher training, I developed something called the traffic light method through a partnership with Dr. Dan Mikeska, a leader in the medical fitness community, to provide some rules of the road to follow during this journey.[22] This traffic light method is fashioned after several well-known fitness safety guidelines, and serves as a simple and easy-to-remember framework for working with clients.

The first step in applying the traffic light method is to review the client's health history, kosha screenings, and interview notes—all of the data we have received from the client thus far. Based on all of the data available, we can then review the wellness continuum (see Figure 7) and pinpoint where we believe the client is on the continuum, to determine if they are in the "red," "yellow," or "green" zone. We can also ask the client to pinpoint where they feel they are on this continuum as well, and discuss whether or not we are in agreement on their location. The client's location on the wellness continuum will then give us a starting point in the design of their one-on-one yoga program, especially with regard to asana. Let's examine what each of these zones can mean for the client's yoga practice and program.

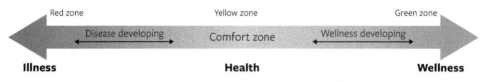

FIGURE 7: THE WELLNESS CONTINUUM[23]

THE RED ZONE—STABILIZING

Clients in the red zone of the wellness continuum likely have compromised physical function and/or are receiving medical care for their condition. They may be experiencing high levels of stress related to their diagnosis and its treatment, and they may also be experiencing side effects from their medications. As a result, we will go slowly with our asana assessments so as to focus on stabilizing the client. We are emphasizing a kapha-inspired practice, celebrating structure and stabilization so as to provide a cooling experience (that isn't inflammatory to their stress of illness, the side effects of their medication, and the illness itself).

THE YELLOW ZONE—CENTERING

Clients in the yellow zone are in what we can call the comfort zone; they are not experiencing difficulty due to illness, but neither are they optimizing their wellness behavior. If a client's data indicates that they are in the yellow zone, we can start in the red zone and introduce yellow zone practices in a cautious and exploratory manner. Here, we focus on centering (physically and mentally), and provide breathwork (pranayama), meditation, and mudras as per the client's needs and program goals. This zone is inspired by pitta dosha, because it aims to both center and stimulate the fire within the client, so they can show up more fully for their wellness journey.

THE GREEN ZONE—MOBILIZING

Clients in the green zone are not experiencing disease and are also taking care of their wellness in an optimal way, focused on prevention. This zone is about enjoying a healthy lifestyle and preventing decline down the continuum. In the Yoga for One asana assessment protocol, we can start with the red zone (stabilizing) and then proceed with caution through the yellow zone (centering). Then, if the client tolerates the yellow zone, we can progress to the green zone, which focuses on mobility and performance. Here we can expand the practice's possibilities, with aims towards strength, flexibility, and cardiovascular and/or balance (neuromuscular facilitation) improvement. A green practice is mostly mat-based practice for asanas to encourage the vata-inspired practice.

Table 3: Overview of the traffic light method

Zone	General intention	What it looks like
Red zone	In the red zone, we take our time to honor our body's needs. In the stillness, we can focus on stabilizing ourselves, and notice how we are moving in the world. We celebrate structure and support, with the chair.	Chair practice Stillness and structure (kapha) Stabilizing the body No sudden movements No extreme temperatures
Yellow zone	After starting in the red zone, we focus on centering ourselves by activating our bandhas and engaging our breath. We slowly mobilize, moving from the center out. And we center our thoughts, choosing to move out of limitation and into self-care.	Chair or mat practice Centering the body Building internal heat (pitta) Moving with spine in mind Moderate breath practices Engagement of bandhas
Green zone	After stabilizing in the red zone and centering in the yellow zone, we can explore how we want to mobilize our strength, flexibility, balance, or cardiovascular health in the practice. We can find freedom to be ourselves in the practice, as we are centered in joy!	Mat practice Mobilizing the body Finding freedom to move (vata) Optimizing fitness (strength, flexibility, cardiovascular, neuromuscular facilitation/ balance)

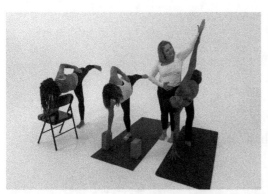
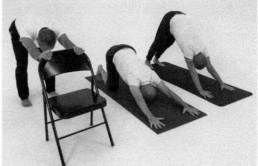
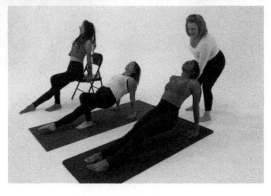

Part 3: Conducting the client asana assessment

ASANA ASSESSMENTS

As you can see, the wellness continuum recognizes that health is more than just the absence of illness; it's a continuous journey towards well-being. Once we determine where the client is on the wellness continuum, we can then decide if we would like to add an asana assessment to our assessment process. If we would like to do so, and the client is agreeable, we can then apply the client's location on the continuum (red, yellow, or green) in our decision-making for conducting the assessment. In other words, the client's current state of illness or wellness will tell us what version of each pose we can practice: red, yellow, or green.

Let's review the asanas I use in my assessment sessions, so you can explore how you can potentially integrate these into your own assessment session. Although every client has their own innate traffic light system (i.e., what is red for one person may be green for another), I share here ways that we can think about the red, yellow, and green zone options. One rule that I generally follow is to use chair poses for the red zone, small props for the yellow zone, and mat-based work in the green zone. As you become more familiar with the traffic light method, you can adapt this approach based on the needs of your clients and your own preferences, as part of your co-creation process.

TADASANA (MOUNTAIN POSE)

Red zone: Foundation and stability

Objective: Establish a stable foundation, moving slow, small, and steady (for stability).

Assessments:

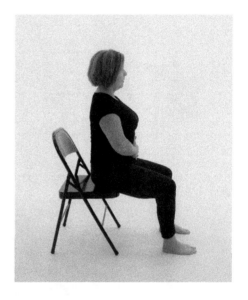

- Ability to get up and out of the chair, and to sit back down with ease

- Postural awareness (Neutral? Kyphotic? Lordotic?)

- Pelvis over middle of foot? (Centered stance)

- Imbalances left or right

- Breath ease vs. lack of ease

- Overall sense of peace, joy, and/or ease.

Yellow zone: Centering and engagement

Objective: Establish core stability for the spine and engage bandhas; centering.

Assessments:

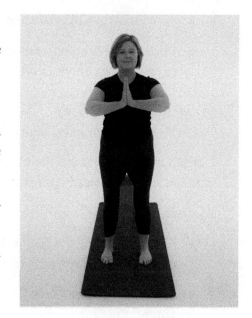

- Ability to engage and hold block with legs (activate core chain from the ground up)

- Centering of neutral spine (uddhyiana bandha)

- Pelvis over middle of foot? (Centered stance)

- Connection with breath.

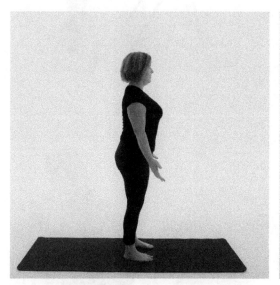
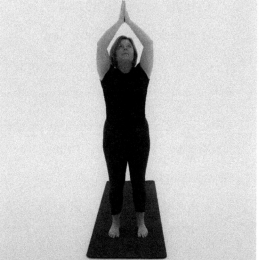

Green zone: Exploration and enhancement

Objective: Mobilize from the center out, optimizing range of motion, strength, stamina, and breath.

Assessments:

- Balance: ability to raise the toes and heels (before coming back to an even stance on the feet).

- Arm flexibility: ability to extend the arms overhead, reaching towards the sky.

- Drishti (gaze direction): explore changing the gaze—looking up, straight ahead, or down. Each offers a different experience in balance and concentration.

UTKATASANA (CHAIR POSE)

Red zone: Foundation and stability

Objective: Establish a stable foundation, moving slow, small, and steady (for stability).

Assessments:

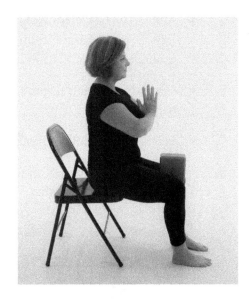

- Ability to get up and out of the chair, and to sit back down with ease

- Postural awareness (Neutral? Kyphotic? Lordotic?)

- Imbalances left or right

- Breath ease vs. lack of ease

- Overall sense of peace, joy, and/or ease.

Yellow zone: Centering and engagement

Objective: Establish core stability for the spine and engage bandhas; centering.

Assessments:

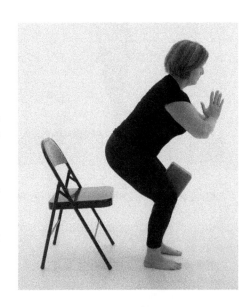

- Ability to engage and hold block with legs (activate core chain from the ground up)

- Centering of neutral spine (uddhyiana bandha)

- Ability to center front body and back body (without going into low back)

- Connection with breath.

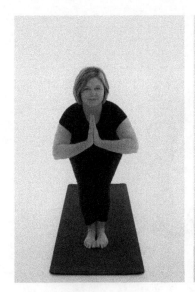 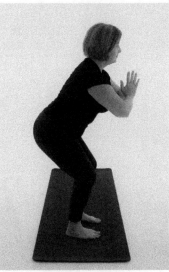 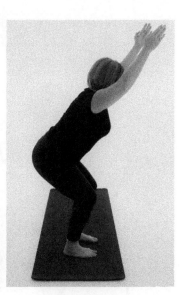

Green zone: Exploration and mobility

Objective: Mobilize from the center out, optimizing range of motion, strength, stamina, and breath.

Assessments:

- Balance: ability to lift onto the balls of the feet, raising the heels off the ground

- Arm flexibility: ability to extend the arms overhead; rotate to sides

- Strength: ability to hold the pose for 3–5 breaths

- Awareness: ability to move in and out from neutral spine.

MARJARYASANA-BITILASANA (CAT–COW POSE)

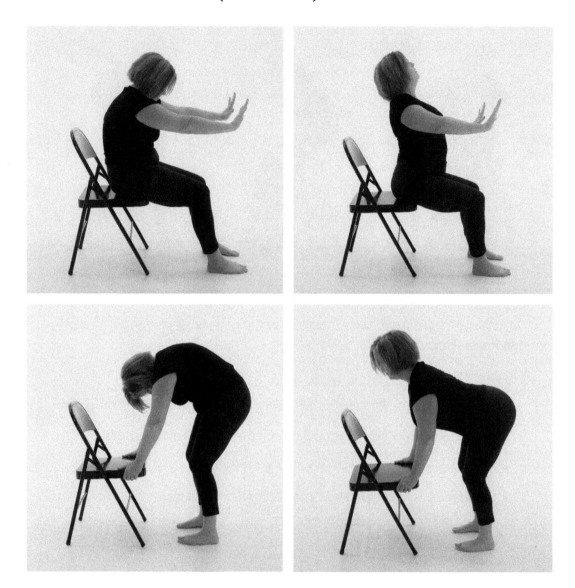

Red zone: Foundation and stability

Objective: Establish a stable foundation, moving slow, small, and steady (for stability).

Assessments:

- Ability to get up and out of the chair, and to sit back down with ease:

  - If can't get out of chair: seated Marjaryasana-Bitilasana

- If can get out of chair: face chair for Marjaryasana-Bitilasana (without going to the floor)

- Spinal awareness: can they move from the center out in their spine?

- Imbalances left or right

- Breath ease vs. lack of ease

- Overall sense of peace, joy, and/or ease.

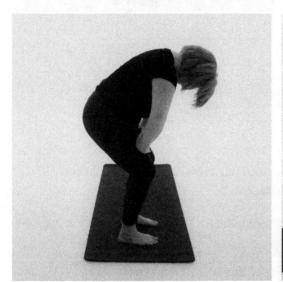 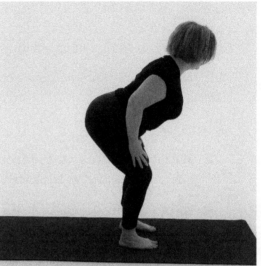

Yellow zone: Centering and engagement

Objective: Establish core stability for the spine and engage bandhas; centering.

Assessments:

- Centering from neutrality in and out of Marjaryasana-Bitilasana without overdoing shoulders

- Ability to center front and back body (without going into low back)

- Connection with breath.

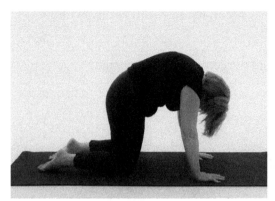 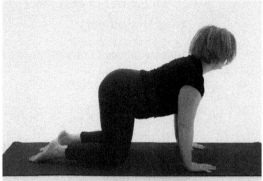

Green zone: Exploration and mobility

Objective: Mobilize from the center out, optimizing range of motion, strength, stamina, and breath.

Assessments:

- Mobility: ability to go to the floor and to put pressure directly on knees. (If this is not possible, go back to yellow zone.)

- Balance: ability to add single leg movement with Marjaryasana-Bitilasana back (tiger)

- Strength: ability to hold the pose for 3–5 breaths

- Awareness: ability to move in and out from neutral spine

- Flexibility: ability to mobilize spine while keeping core control lumbar and cervical.

ADHO MUKHA SVANASANA (DOWNWARD FACING DOG)

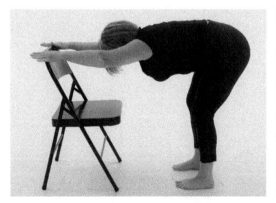 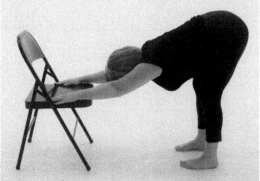

Red zone: Foundation and stability

Objective: Establish a stable foundation, moving slow, small, and steady (for stability).

Assessments:

- Ability to get up and out of the chair, and to sit back down with ease:
  - If the client can't get out of the chair, raise arms overhead (not pictured)
  - If the client can get out of the chair, face the chair for a gentle stretch with head even with heart, progressing to head lower than heart

- Spinal awareness: can they move from the center out in their spine?

- Imbalances left or right

- Breath ease vs. lack of ease

- Overall sense of peace, joy, and/or ease.

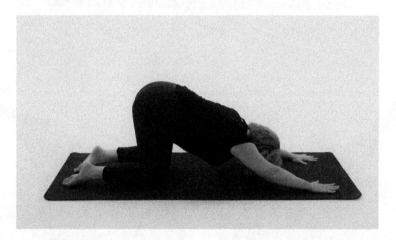

Yellow zone: Centering and engagement

Objective: Establish core stability for the spine and engage bandhas; centering.

Assessments:

- Ability to go to floor:
  - If yes, go to the floor and set up for Uttana Shishoasana (Puppy-Downward Facing Dog) with knees on the floor
  - If no, go back to red zone variation with the chair

- Centering from neutrality in and out of the posture

- Ability to center front body and back body (without going into low back)

- Flexibility: ability to raise arms overhead and take shoulders into deep flexion without raising shoulders (side body flexibility and shoulder flexibility)

- Connection with breath.

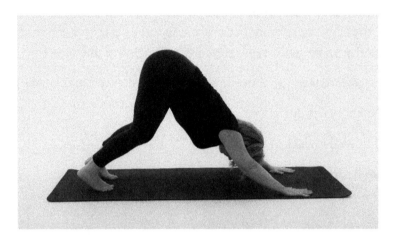

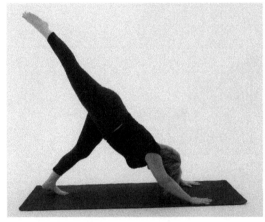
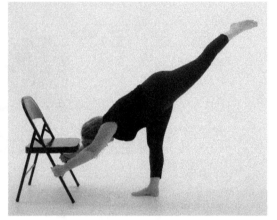

Green zone: Exploration and mobility

Objective: Mobilize from the center out, optimizing range of motion, strength, stamina, and breath.

Assessments:

- Balance: ability to be upside down (inversion); add single-legged Adho Mukha Svanasana

- Strength: ability to hold the pose for 3–5 breaths

- Awareness: ability to move in and out from neutral spine

- Flexibility: ability to lengthen legs (work towards unbending the knees) without rounding the low back.

VIRABHADRASANA II (WARRIOR 2) AND VIPARITA VIRABHADRASANA (REVERSE WARRIOR)

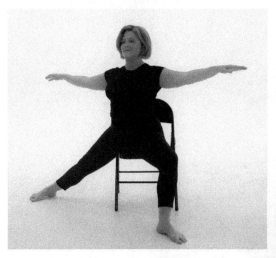
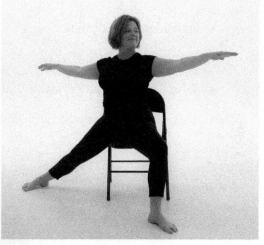

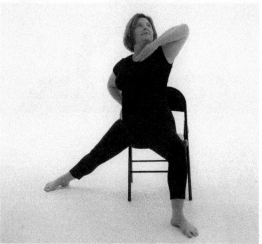

Red zone: Foundation and stability

Objective: Establish a stable foundation, moving slow, small, and steady (for stability).

Assessments:

- Ability to get up and out of the chair, and to sit back down with ease:

  - If the client can't get out of the chair: seated facing the corner; legs in front
  - If the client can get out of the chair: stand next to the chair and use the back for balance support (not pictured)

- Hip flexibility: can they rotate the long leg side internally (keeping the knee in alignment with toes) and the bent leg side externally (keeping knee above ankle)?

- Imbalances left or right

- Breath ease vs. lack of ease

- Overall sense of peace, joy, and/or ease

- Flexibility: side body and shoulder.

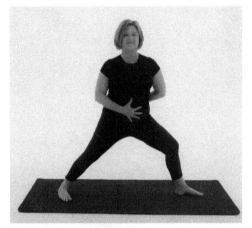

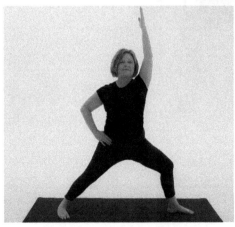
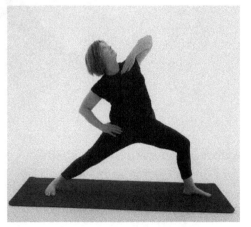

Yellow zone: Centering and engagement

Objective: Establish core stability for the spine and engage bandhas; centering.

Assessments:

- Ability to stay centered and elongated in neutral spine between Marjaryasana and Bitilasana (Cat and Cow Pose)

- Ability to raise arm to side (lateral stretch)

- Ability to take torso to either side (lateral flexion)

- Ability to use core control to maintain neutrality in and out of poses, and protect neck

- Connection with breath.

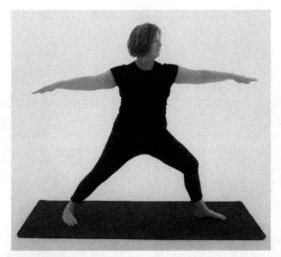

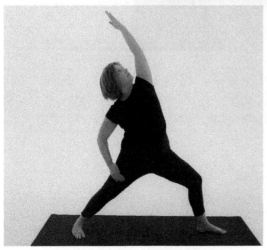

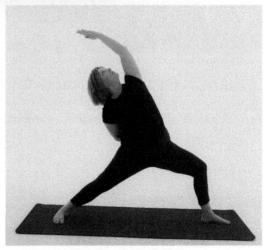

Green zone: Exploration and mobility

Objective: Mobilize from the center out, optimizing range of motion, strength, stamina, and breath.

Assessments:

- Balance: ability to stay steady even when going into Viparita Virabhadrasana

- Strength: ability to hold the pose for 3–5 breaths

- Awareness: ability to rotate from the hips without going into the low back

- Flexibility: can they rotate their hip on the long leg side internally (keeping the knee in alignment with toes without rolling the ankle) and the bent leg side externally (keeping knee above ankle and not past the toes)?

VRKSASANA (TREE POSE)

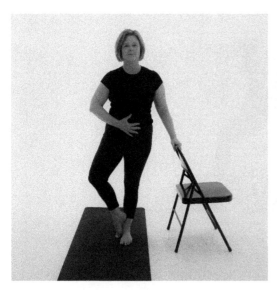 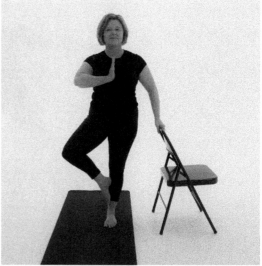

Red zone: Foundation and stability

Objective: Establish a stable foundation, moving slow, small, and steady (for stability).

Assessments:

- Ability to stand:
  - If the client can't get out of the chair: stay seated in the chair and engage in gentle hip opener (not pictured)

- – If the client can get out of the chair: stand next to the chair and hold on to the back for support

- Ability to balance:

   - – If the client is unable to balance themselves on one leg into a mostly steady state, keep both feet on the ground
   - – If the client is able to balance steadily on one leg, take the raised leg to a comfortable position and continue to use the wall or chair for support

- Imbalances left or right

- Breath ease vs. lack of ease

- Overall sense of peace, joy, and/or ease

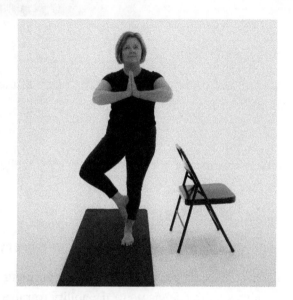

Yellow zone: Centering and engagement

Objective: Establish core stability for the spine and engage bandhas; centering.

Assessment:

- Awareness of hips during foot raise

- Ability to balance in the pose with one foot off the floor and take hands off the chair

- Exploration of subtle body movements like slightly closing the eyes or introducing gentle breath practices to enhance focus.

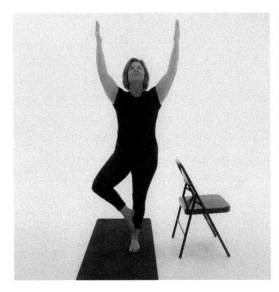 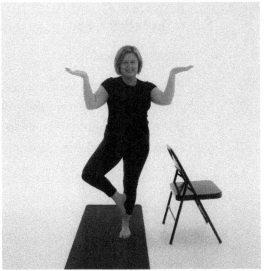

Green zone: Exploration and mobility

Objective: Mobilize from the center out, optimizing range of motion, strength, stamina, and breath.

Assessments:

- Balance: ability to stay steady in the lower body even while mobilizing the upper body

- Strength: ability to hold the pose for 3–5 breaths

- Awareness: ability to keep hips even and raise arms; close eyes (optional)

- Flexibility: ability to raise the foot up the leg to the perineum (not pictured) while keeping hips square (pelvis neutral); ability to raise arms overhead without raising or rounding shoulders.

PARSVA BALASANA (BIRD DOG POSE)

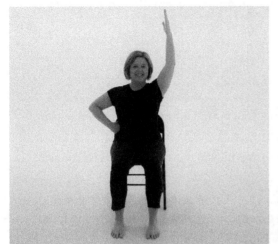
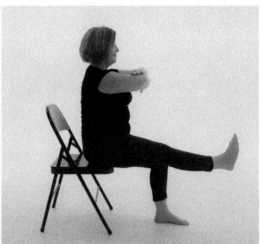

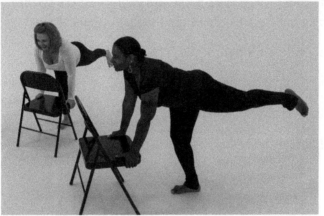

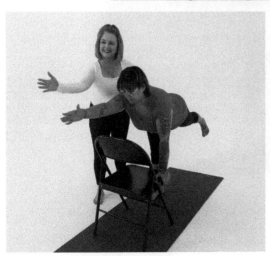
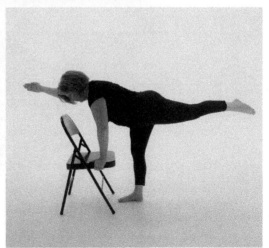

Red zone: Foundation and stability

Objective: Establish a stable foundation, moving slow, small, and steady (for stability).

Assessments:

- Ability to get off the chair:

    - If the client can't get off the chair: stay seated and work arms and legs in opposition
    - If the client can get to the chair: turn and face the chair; use the chair seat

- Ability to balance (stand on one leg):

    - If the client can't stand on one leg, keep them seated in the chair and focus on moving limbs in opposition
    - If the client can stand on one leg: explore where the arms can be while keeping torso square (hips and shoulders aligned)

- Imbalances left or right

- Breath ease vs. lack of ease

- Overall sense of peace, joy, and/or ease

- Flexibility: side body and shoulder.

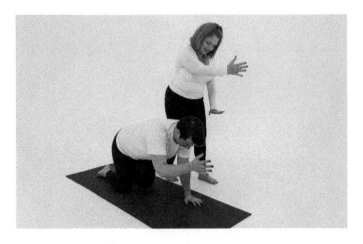

Yellow zone: Centering and engagement

Objective: Establish core stability for the spine and engage bandhas; centering.

Assessment:

- Awareness of torso "square" during arm and leg raises (staying neutral)

- Ability to balance with one arm reaching forward and opposite leg reaching backward

- Exploration of subtle body movements like slightly closing the eyes or introducing gentle breath practices to enhance focus.

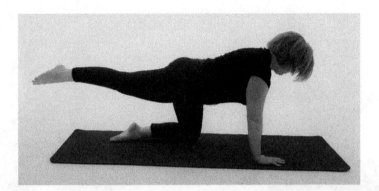

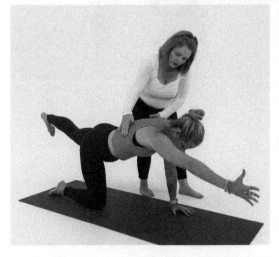 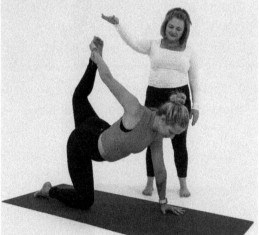

Green zone: Exploration and mobility

Objective: Mobilize from the center out, optimizing range of motion, strength, stamina, and breath.

Assessments:

- Balance: ability to reach forward while maintaining steadiness

- Strength: ability to hold the pose for 3–5 breaths

- Awareness: ability to use opposite arm and leg

- Flexibility: ability to lengthen leg into hip extension without arching low back; ability to flex (reach) shoulder without rounding upper torso.

PARSVA BALASANA (THREAD THE NEEDLE POSE)

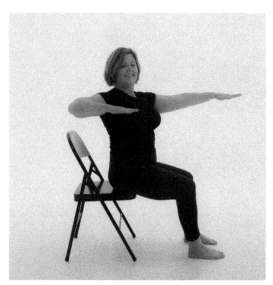 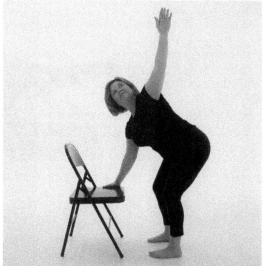

Red zone: Foundation and stability

Objective: Establish a stable foundation, moving slow, small, and steady (for stability).

Assessments:

- Ability to get off the chair:

  - If the client can't get off the chair: stay seated and move torso to either side (arms in the air)
  - If the client can get off the chair: turn and face the chair; use the chair seat for hand anchor

- Imbalances left or right

- Breath ease vs. lack of ease

- Overall sense of peace, joy, and/or ease.

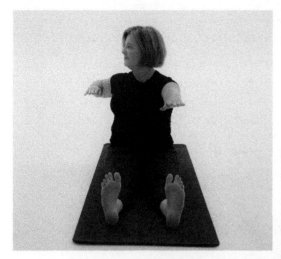
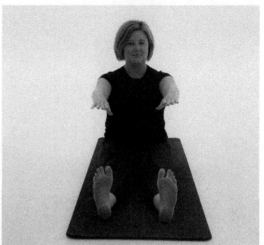
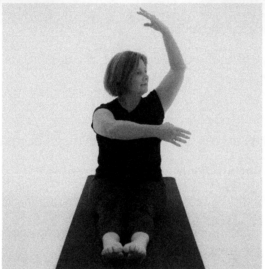

Yellow zone: Centering and engagement

Objective: Establish core stability for the spine and engage bandhas; centering.

Assessment:

- Awareness of torso "square" during arm and leg raises (staying neutral)
- Ability to balance with one arm reaching outward and upward.

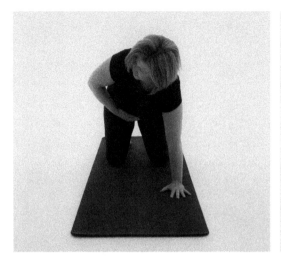 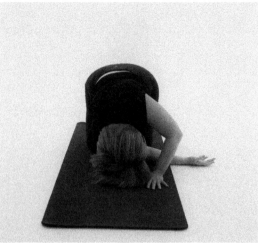

Green zone: Exploration and mobility

Objective: Mobilize from the center out, optimizing range of motion, strength, stamina, and breath.

Assessments:

- Balance: ability to keep hips even while rotating side to side

- Strength: ability to hold the pose for 3–5 breaths

- Awareness: ability to keep scapulohumeral rhythm in sync

- Flexibility: rotation ability side to side; ability to raise arm while turning outwardly (not pictured).

DANDASANA (PLANK POSE)

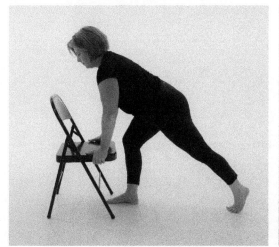 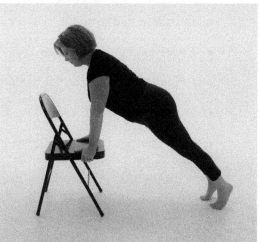

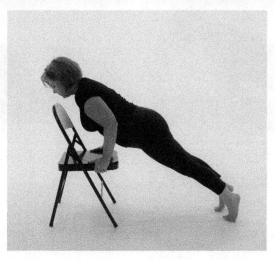

Red zone: Foundation and stability

Objective: Establish a stable foundation, moving slow, small, and steady (for stability).

Assessments:

- Ability to get off the chair:

  - If the client can't get off the chair: stay seated and move arms in the air (not pictured)

- If the client can get off the chair: turn and face the chair; try lunges (one leg of support), then full dandasana (both legs back)

- Imbalances left or right

- Breath ease vs. lack of ease

- Overall sense of peace, joy, and/or ease

- Flexibility: wrists

- Upper body strength: ability to hold Dandasana; Chaturanga (Low Plank) (optional).

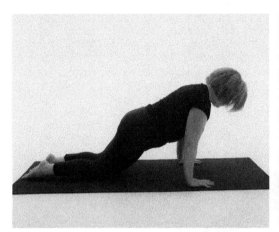 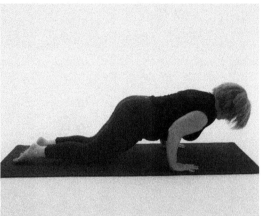

Yellow zone: Centering and engagement

Objective: Establish core stability for the spine and engage bandhas; centering.

Assessment:

- Awareness of torso "square" during Dandasana (staying neutral)

- Ability to hold the posture with core control and steady breath.

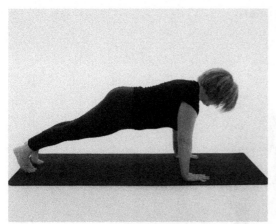
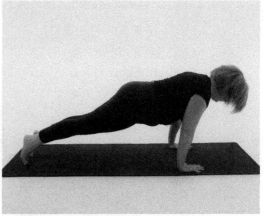
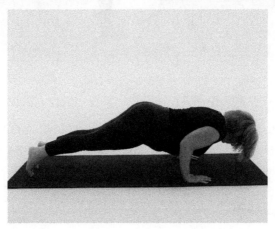

Green zone: Exploration and mobility

Objective: Mobilize from the center out, optimizing range of motion, strength, stamina, and breath.

Assessments:

- Balance: ability to stay neutral and even on both sides (not go into low back)

- Strength: ability to hold the pose for 3–5 breaths; ability to keep shoulder blades stable without "winging scapulae" (engage serratus anterior not rhomboids)

- Awareness: ability to stack elbows over wrists; maintain elbows in Chaturanga (Low Plank)

- Flexibility: wrist flexibility (hands with palms fully on mat); hip flexor flexibility.

SETU BANDHA SARVANGASANA (BRIDGE POSE)

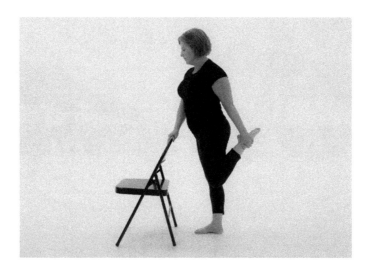

Red zone: Foundation and stability

Objective: Establish a stable foundation, moving slow, small, and steady (for stability).

Assessments:

- Ability to get to the floor:
  - If can't get to the floor, try standing quad stretch
  - Carefully explore if holding on is necessary

- Imbalances left or right

- Breath ease vs. lack of ease

- Overall sense of peace, joy, and/or ease

- Flexibility: ability to lengthen hip flexors with knee under pelvis and low back neutral; ability to reach shoulder back into extension (behind torso).

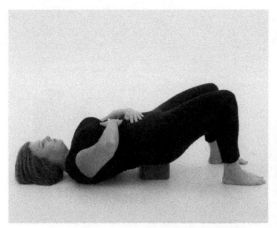
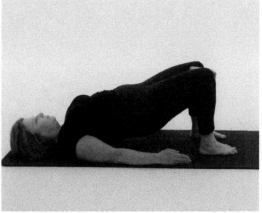
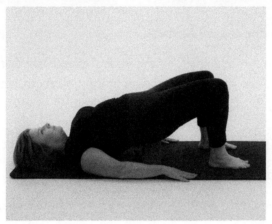

Yellow zone: Centering and engagement

Objective: Establish core stability for the spine and engage bandhas; centering.

Assessment:

- Awareness of feet in alignment with hips
- Ability to articulate spine up and down vs. move from neutral spine
- Ability to hold the block between the thighs
- Movement ability to move arms opposite to hips.

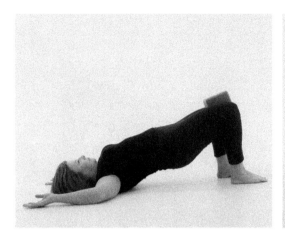 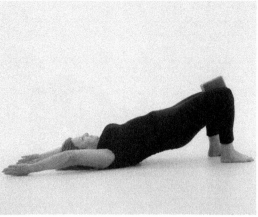

Green zone: Centering and engagement

Objective: Establish core stability for the spine and engage bandhas; centering. Mobilize from the center out, optimizing range of motion, strength, stamina, and breath.

Assessments:

- Balance: ability to stay neutral and even on both sides (not go into low back)

- Strength: ability to hold the pose for 3–5 breaths

- Awareness: ability to stack elbows over wrists; maintain elbows in Chaturanga (Low Plank)

- Flexibility: wrist flexibility (hands with palms fully on mat); hip flexor flexibility.

SAVASANA (RELAXATION POSE)

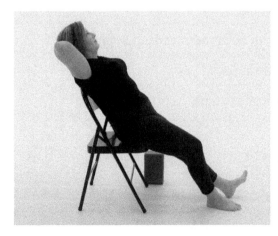 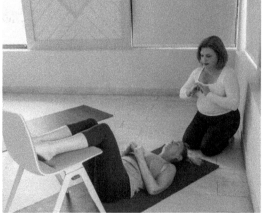

Red zone: Foundation and stability

Objective: Establish a stable foundation, moving slow, small, and steady (for stability).

Assessments:

- Overall sense of peace, joy, and/or ease

- Comfort: do they need a blanket? Pillow? Prop?

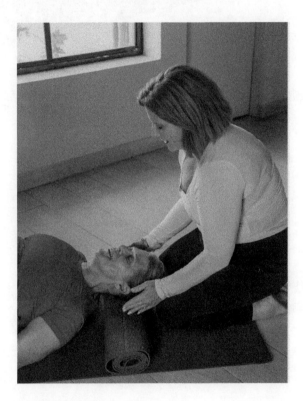

Yellow zone: Centering and engagement

Objective: Establish core stability for the spine and engage bandhas; centering.

Assessment:

- Awareness of need for support

- Need for support for head and/or knees, helping the client to find as close to neutral spine as is comfortable for their body.

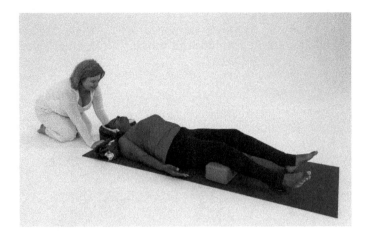

Green zone: Exploration and mobility

Objective: Ability to relax and enjoy stillness.

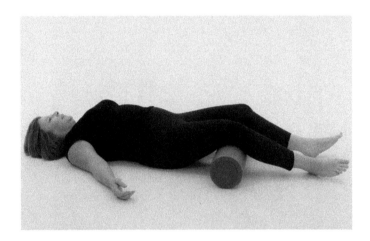

Assessment session mind–body scan: somatic sensory meditation

After leading the client through the intake process (pre-sessions), interview (to determine their unique situation and goals), and assessment session (to review their practice of asanas), I like to lead the client through a mind–body scan. This serves two purposes. First, it gives the client a moment of transition between the session and the rest of their day through a somatic practice. Second, I can watch the client's comfort level during the mind–body scan to see how ready they are for further meditation work.

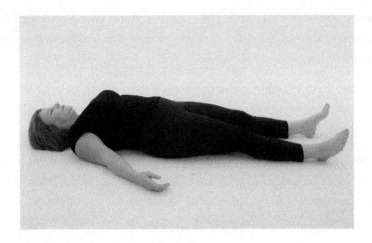

Part 1: Guidance

Begin by finding a quiet and comfortable place to sit or lie down. Close your eyes if you feel comfortable doing so, and take a few deep breaths to relax.

- *Body awareness:* Start by bringing your attention to your body. Feel the weight of your body pressing into the chair or the ground beneath you. Take a moment to notice any sensations in your body, without judgment. These sensations could include warmth, coolness, tension, or relaxation. Simply observe them.

- *Breath awareness:* Shift your focus to your breath. Feel the natural rhythm of your breath as it moves in and out of your body. Notice the rise and fall of your chest and abdomen as you breathe. Be fully present with each breath, feeling the sensations of the breath as it enters and leaves your body.

- *Progressive relaxation:* Starting at the top of your head, slowly scan your body down to your toes. As you do, bring your awareness to each part of your body. As you focus on each part, notice any sensations you feel there. It could be warmth, tingling, tension, or relaxation. Simply observe without trying to change anything. If you notice any tension or discomfort in any area, imagine your breath flowing into that area, helping to release any tension or discomfort.

- *Sensory exploration:* Now bring your attention to your sense of touch. Notice the sensation of the clothes against your skin or any other sensations on your skin. Pay attention to the feeling of the air against your skin. Feel the temperature and any subtle movements in the air around you.

- *Sound awareness:* Tune in to the sounds around you. Notice any sounds in your environment, whether they are near or distant. Simply observe them without judgment.

- *Smell and taste:* Take a moment to notice if there are any scents or tastes in the air. Whether it's a subtle aroma or the taste of your own breath, be present with these sensations.

- *Whole body awareness:* Gradually expand your awareness to encompass your entire body as a whole. Feel the entirety of your body, from head to toe. Imagine your whole body being filled with a sense of calm and relaxation. Allow any tension to melt away as you continue to breathe deeply.

- *Gratitude:* Take a moment to express gratitude for your body and its ability to experience these sensations. Be thankful for this moment of mindfulness.

- *Closing:* When you're ready, gently bring your awareness back to your breath. Take a few deep breaths, and slowly begin to wiggle your fingers and toes.

- *Open your eyes:* When you feel ready, open your eyes and reorient yourself to the present moment.

Part 2: Reflection

After reflecting on your experience, please share with me...

How did this experience go for you, generally?

- What specifically did you notice?
- Can you describe any or all of the following:
  - Self-awareness?
  - Thoughts?
  - Feelings?
  - Sensory experience?

CONCLUSION

Through these first four of the five steps of SOAP, we have applied an evidence-informed approach. By listening to the client's story and supporting them in sense-making, we have prioritized their lived experience (the first "E" of the evidence-informed practice). By requesting the client's completion of health history forms and screening tools in alignment with their desired program goals, we have collected evidence (formative data) of their current sense-making situation and priorities for their Yoga for One program and practice design. And, by reviewing data collected in Steps 1 through 3, and using this to make informed choices in how we assess the client in the asana assessment session, we have applied our training and expertise into the co-creation process.

In the next chapter we will continue the journey through the fifth step of the SOAP process, by focusing on program and practice planning. Here we will continue with our commitment to stay inclusive and to an evidence-informed process, in the co-creation of a yoga program.

CHAPTER 6

Co-Creating an Evidence-Informed Program Plan

In the 1980s a professor introduced me to the following quote from Benjamin Franklin:

> If you are failing to plan, you are planning to fail...

It has stuck with me ever since. Although I recognize that the terms "failing" and "fail" may be a little harsh for those of us who are yoga professionals, I share this quote to start off this chapter because I want to emphasize the important role that planning ahead has in any venture—including the co-creation of a yoga practice program.

In this chapter I will share how you can plan out a yoga program that supports clients both on and off the mat. You'll see how we can take the concepts we have learned about co-creation, inclusivity, and shared decision-making, and apply them to our work with clients. This chapter focuses on how you can use logic modeling (a simple planning technique that we use in the practice of public health when designing enterprise-level health campaigns) to co-create a Yoga for One practice program.

LET'S BRING ORDER INTO CHAOS...WITH STRATEGIC PLANNING AND EVALUATION

Did you know that you engage in program planning and evaluation every day? Every time you think about where you want to go, why you want to go there, choose how and when you'll make it happen, and track your progress along the way, you are engaging in a program planning and evaluation process.

The *strategic planning process* includes all the steps that are necessary to build out your plan (or road map) for your client. The plan illustrates the path of how you will get to where you want to go tomorrow, based on where you are today. As mentioned in Chapter 5, the evaluation and assessment processes serve as your GPS navigation system, helping you to know where you are relative to where you want to be (assessment) and how well you are doing relative to your plans (evaluation).

You wouldn't want to begin a journey without a road map—otherwise you wouldn't know where you are going or how you will get there. And you wouldn't want to leave home without a map or GPS, because you might find yourself in the middle of the trip feeling lost somewhere between where you started and where you hope to finish—having no idea how to get back on track to the map's plan. In a similar way, the strategic planning, evaluation, and assessment processes work together to ensure that the plan is both strategic and realistic.

For this reason, I invite you to join me in using strategic planning and evaluation processes in the co-creation of a one-on-one yoga program. In this way you can ensure that your client's programs and practices are not just "going nowhere"—but instead, are supporting them in going from where they are today (in their current challenges) and supporting them in going where they want to go (to their desired future state of health, wellness, and well-being).

INTRODUCING...LOGIC MODELING FOR PROGRAM DESIGN (AND CO-CREATION)

In the field of program planning and evaluation, a *logic model*, also known as a *program logic model* or *theory of change*, is a visual representation (framework) that illustrates the logical connections between the various components of a program, project, or intervention. I have found in my research and my practice work that logic models offer us one big picture view of the program. They give us a simple, scientific, and straightforward way to co-create the program concept, through the use of graphics. They serve as a communication tool, helping us to ensure that we and our clients are literally "on the same page" with our shared decision-making in the process of co-creating the program. And they offer the following additional benefits:

- Provide all stakeholders (including the client) with a plan (road map)

- Guide facilitation of the decision-making pathway (i.e., conversation guide)

- Build trust and rapport as a "team-building" (partnership) exercise

- Clarify and document decisions made during the shared decision-making process

- Promote understanding of the program for all stakeholders, with a "big picture" view of the key components of a program

- Define the intended outcomes and impacts of a program, to understand its "why"

- Articulate program goals and objectives to describe and measure success

- Identify key activities and resources (inputs) required to make the program happen

- Synchronize program planning, evaluation, assessment, monitoring, and reporting efforts

- Ensure that all key components of a program have their own strategy, and that there is an overarching strategy for the program as a whole.

You, too, can become an implementation scientist!

As noted by Pearson *et al.* (2020),[24] logic models are a best practice in the field of *implementation science*—a multi-disciplinary field that focuses on understanding the methods, strategies, and processes for effectively integrating evidence-based and evidence-informed interventions or programs into real-world settings. Implementation science seeks to bridge the gap between research evidence and real-world practice by examining how best to launch, implement, and scale practices and programs.

The primary goal of implementation science is to generate knowledge and evidence about what does and doesn't work in the process of implementing an intervention—and why this is the case. Implementation scientists (like me, and now you!) focus the majority of their attention on the development of strategies and approaches that enhance the adoption, sustainability, and fidelity of evidence-based and evidence-informed programs.

This book is an example of an implementation science effort, because I am aiming to equip you with the knowledge you need to bridge the gap between research and the real world—in your own realistic way. I also hope that you will take this knowledge and transform it into your own know-how—so that you, too, can become an implementation scientist when you partner with those receiving care to co-create their one-on-one yoga practice program.

I have been honored to co-create logic models with individual clients, teams, organizations, and government agencies (in the USA and globally). I will share with you here what I have learned about how we can create them swiftly and well—which is both a process to follow as well as a skill to develop over time. Like any new tool it may take you some time to get used to using it, but once you do, I believe (based on my past experience and current work) that you will find it a helpful way to co-create practice programs in a person-centered way.

What is included in the Yoga for One logic model?

A logic model typically has a group of key components—which you might think of as steps in an overall journey. Here are the components that I like to include in the logic model design process (aka, logic modeling) (see Figure 8):

- *Priorities:* A list of problems that the effort (in this case, the program) seeks to solve.

- *Inputs/resources:* The resources, such as funding, staff, facilities, or equipment, invested in the program.

- *Activities:* The specific actions or interventions undertaken as part of the program. These can include services provided, workshops conducted, or strategies implemented.

- *Outputs:* The direct products or deliverables of the program activities. These are often quantitative and measurable, such as the number of participants trained, the number of events held, or the materials distributed.

- *Outcomes:* The short-term, intermediate, or long-term changes that result from the program. Outcomes are typically categorized into three levels: short term (changes in knowledge, attitudes, or behavior), intermediate (changes in skills or conditions), and long term (changes in social, economic, or environmental conditions).

- *Vision and impact:* The ultimate desired effect or broader social change that the program aims to achieve. Impacts are often related to improved quality of life, increased equity, or enhanced well-being at the individual, community, or societal level.

As we will see, these steps make sense when we take a look at them in chronological order—from priorities to vision. However, we do not build a logic model in this order; instead, we start with our desired future state (vision for success), and then work backwards. In this way, we are choosing our final destination for our journey, and then mapping out the path to get there. When we go about the actual travel of the journey (enactment of the plan), we start at the beginning. For this reason, many logic model geeks like me often say, "Build the logic model right to left, but live it left to right."

In our Yoga for One practice program efforts, *I recommend that we, as yoga professionals, engage in shared decision-making to co-create the logic model.* As we partner with the person receiving care (the client), we avoid building out "cookie-cutter" programs that may or may not be relevant for the person/s they are delivered to. Rather than creating a one-size-fits-all program without the inputs from the people it is meant to serve, I recommend that we co-create a one-of-a-kind program for one client at a time by involving them throughout the logic modeling process.

Through the practice of shared decision-making (described in Chapter 2) we can co-create the logic model, step by step, and support the client in making choices for each logic model category (component). The plan (road map) emerges on the page before our eyes as we document the results of each shared decision made for each of the logic model components. Through this process, the client has the ability to "see their thinking" on the page in front of them, while we are also documenting the details of their program plan and evaluation process. Once we have moved through the decisions that need to be made for each component, we can then take a step back to look at the logic model overall as a big picture. Here, we can again engage in shared decision-making, to explore with the client if the logic model does or doesn't work for them—within each component and as a whole.

During the conversations that occur in the processes of shared decision-making and co-creation, both the yoga facilitator and the client are learning more about each other's perspectives, assumptions, and beliefs, while also learning if they are on the same program "page" (i.e., plan or map). Sometimes in this process it is revealed that there are two entirely different pages going on for the yoga facilitator and the client. If there is discord or disconnect between the yoga facilitator and the client, the co-creation process can't continue—because you can't be on two maps (roads) at the same time.

In summary, logic models provide us with an overall road map for a program. In the ideal scenario, we partner with the client to co-create them, and involve other key stakeholders in the decision-making process too.

How can we use the Yoga for One logic model template to describe the program?

As you facilitate the client's decision-making with the logic model, please remember to stay grounded so that you can hold non-judgmental, healing presence for them. We want to encourage them to not only make decisions, but to also notice what comes up within them as they do so. There will be times when the questions are uncomfortable, or the answers are hard to admit to. We can maintain steadfastness for the client, by practicing healing presence and holding them in positive regard. If we find that their discomfort is beyond our scope of practice, we need to refer them to another allied health professional or emergency services if they show severe signs of duress. It is our responsibility to stay within our scope of practice while also stewarding them to the support that they need for their safety and well-being, across the entire wellness continuum.

As you can see in Figure 8, the logic model has six sections, each with their own series of considerations for the Yoga for One program (Priorities, Inputs, Activities, Outputs, Outcomes, and Impact). In the following process, I will show you how you can build out the logic model for each individual client, using a step-by-step process.

Step 1: Set the vision (choose the desired destination)

Here, in the first step of the co-creation process of the yoga practice program, we support the client in setting the ideal vision they have for their program's success. Much like you choose a destination for a journey, here the client is encouraged to choose the vision they want to focus on for the program. Although every client needs a different type of customized support in the visioning process, I have found in my private practice that the following questions can help them to create a vision that isn't just about them individually—but one that also connects them to their greater sense of purpose in their life (interpersonally) and in the world (societally), in keeping with the socio-ecological model.

YOGA FOR ONE VISION-SETTING QUESTIONS

The following questions are designed to support you in creating a vision for your customized yoga program. Please use a journal to either write out a response to the following questions, and/or draw a picture of your vision for each question. Since yoga is ultimately a practice of self-realization and self-liberation, this is an opportunity to articulate your vision of what a life of joy could look like for you; one that connects your own sense of self-liberation with your ability to connect in your relationships and your ability to show up in service to the world. Now is the time to allow yourself to dream big, as though you had a magic wand that could make anything possible! (We will work on how you can head towards your vision through the program in later steps.)

Part 1: My Vision for My Self (Self-Self)
Here you are invited to illustrate the theme of self-liberation, in words and/or a picture. What could a life of "freedom to be yourself" look like and feel for you?

Part 2: My Vision for Connection in Relationships (Self-Others)
Here you are invited to illustrate the theme of connection, in words and/or a picture. What could a life of shared support (both given and received) look like and feel for you?

Part 3: My Vision for My Service to the World (Self-Others)
Here you are invited to illustrate the theme of Service. This can be thought of in serving above self (for a greater good), and/or a sense of service to a higher calling (tapping into your spiritual belief system). What could a life of Service to something bigger than yourself look like and feel for you?

After reflecting on your answers to these questions, I invite you to notice any themes that have already come up in your vision for program success. How would you now describe your vision of your future state? Please feel free to answer this question with words, a non-verbal gesture, and/or by drawing a picture to visualize what your vision of your future state looks like for you.

Step 1	Step 2	Step 3	Step 4	Step 5	Step 6
VISION AND IMPACT	**PRIORITIES**	**OUTCOMES**	**OUTPUTS**	**ACTIVITIES**	**INPUTS**
Envision "There"	**Define "Here"**	**Set Milestones**	**Select Measures**	**Map the Journey**	**Prepare and Pack**
Begin the Yoga for One program planning process by asking the client to describe their vision for their Yoga for One program. Then ask them to share how they foresee that program success will impact: • Themselves (self-liberation) • Relationships (connection) • Greater Good (Service/Dharma)	Ask the client to complete their intake forms and conduct a sense-making interview to learn more about their lived experience. Then, complete additional assessments and/or a literature review to enhance your objective (professional) understanding. Then, collaborate with the client to define their top program priorities.	Consider how long the client's road is from "here" (priorities) to "there" (vision). Then, create a road map of short-, mid- and long-term goals and discuss together how you can make these goals SMART: • Specific • Measurable • Achievable • Relevant • Time-Bound	Ask the client for permission to measure success. If they agree, ask them how they would describe success for the program's short-, mid- and long-term goals. Then, partner with the client to decide how you will measure their progress for each goal and for the program overall—before, during and after the program.	Within your professional scope of practice, draw a program "journey map" of activities (program tactics) that will take your client from "here" to "there". The program map may include but not be limited to: • Yoga philosophy • Yoga practices • Yoga postures • Lifestyle change Revise based on client feedback.	Once the journey is mapped out, ask the client to reflect on their readiness to take the program journey. Do they have the resources and readiness they need to succeed throughout the program journey? If Yes: Start the program journey! If No: Repeat Steps 1-6

FIGURE 8: YOGA FOR ONE PROGRAM LOGIC MODEL

Step 2: "Establish our location" (prioritize today's challenges)

Here, in the second step of the co-creation process of your yoga practice program, we go back to the beginning of the program—which is where we are today. You might say we are identifying your current location so we can compare how close we are today to your program's final destination—the vision we explored in Step 1 of where you want to go tomorrow. There are six areas we can explore in this section. Let's explore them, and then I will ask you to reflect on which area/s you want to prioritize, and how you want to prioritize them.

Health and wellness

Where are you on the health and wellness continuum, as shown in Figure 7?

Based on where you are today, what would you say is your priority?

- Protection (I want to stay where I am)?

- Prevention (I don't want to slide left or backwards)?

- Promotion (I want to keep moving forward in a healthy direction)?

World Health Organization Five Well-Being Index (WHO-5)

Based on your answers to the WHO-5, what area of well-being would you like to prioritize (focus on improving) in your yoga program:

- "I have felt cheerful and in good spirits" = emotional well-being (anandamaya kosha)

- "I have felt active and vigorous" = physical well-being (annamaya kosha)

- "I have felt calm and relaxed" = mental well-being (manomaya kosha)

- "I woke up feeling refreshed and rested" = social well-being (pranamaya kosha)

- "My daily life has been filled with things that interest me" = purpose well-being (vijnanamaya kosha)

Social determinants of health

We know that the social determinants of health play an important role in the success of any yoga program plan. Based on your answers to the social determinants of health survey, what determinants do you think could help you find success in your program? What determinants do you feel may make success difficult?

Lifestyle medicine

Lifestyle medicine is a dynamic and evidence-based approach that emphasizes the impact of lifestyle choices on our health and vitality. It recognizes that factors such as nutrition, physical activity, sleep, stress management, and social connections play a pivotal role in our overall well-being. Based on your answers to the lifestyle medicine survey, what lifestyle factors do you want to include or focus on in your yoga program?

Doshas and gunas

Incorporating the ancient wisdom of Ayurveda and yogic philosophy, the concepts of doshas and gunas offer profound insights into our constitution and character, helping us understand our unique physical, mental, and emotional tendencies. Doshas (vata, pitta, and kapha) provide a framework for understanding our innate qualities, while gunas (sattva, rajas, and tamas) shed light on the nature of our mind and emotions. By gaining clarity about your dosha composition, and recognizing prevalent gunas in your life, you'll gain valuable insights into the ways you can tailor your yoga practice and lifestyle choices for maximum well-being. Based on your answers to your doshas and gunas, what do you want to include or focus on in your yoga program?

Koshas

The koshas represent the five sheaths or layers that envelop the human being, ranging from the physical to the subtle. These include annamaya kosha (the physical body), pranamaya kosha (the energy or vital body), manomaya kosha (the mental body), vijnanamaya kosha (the wisdom or intellectual body), and anandamaya kosha (the bliss sheath). Identifying one of these koshas as the priority focus for a one-on-one yoga program is pivotal for several reasons. First, it allows for a personalized and tailored approach, addressing the specific layer that requires attention and enhancement in the individual's life. Second, by honing in on a particular kosha, the yoga program can be structured to provide a profound and holistic transformation, catering to the individual's unique needs and aspirations. Ultimately, this approach empowers the individual to delve deep into their being, fostering a sense of self-awareness and self-realization, which are fundamental goals of yoga practice. In essence, the identification of a kosha as a priority focus serves as the compass guiding the yoga program towards a more profound and meaningful journey of self-discovery and well-being.

Steps 1 and 2 wrap up: choose your top two priorities (yoga on and off the mat)

Although all of these dimensions are relevant for your yoga practice program, it is important to choose your top priorities for your program. I like to think of this as yoga on and off the mat—supporting clients in deciding what one goal they would like to achieve off the mat (in the ways they are practicing lifestyle medicine, or dinacharya), and one goal they would like to achieve on the mat (through daily sadhana—yoga practices, postures, and/or study of philosophy). The mat is a metaphor for the individual's life on the outside (in the world) and life on the inside (in their koshas). Although yoga is really a practice of self-liberation that aims to help individuals to achieve connection within themselves—at the deep layers of the vijnanamaya and anandamaya koshas—it also helps individuals to consider how their life in the world and how their life within themselves needs to change. This is the "location" they want to leave, in order to find a brighter day in their vision of success.

Steps 3 and 4: Set SMART outcome goals and outputs—"Map out the milestones"

In Steps 3 and 4 of Yoga for One program planning and evaluation, we begin the process of co-creating the road map that will take you and your client from where you are today (priorities) to where you would like to be (vision of impact). As you'll see, it's important to conduct Steps 3 and 4 together, as part of this planning process.

In Step 3, we define the goals, or outcomes, we would like to achieve in the program. In Step 4, we decide how we will measure the outputs, or results, of our efforts towards making this change. Together these two steps enable us to create goals that are "SMART":

- *Specific:* For example, instead of setting a broad outcome goal of "I want to manage stress," we can set a more specific one such as "I want to take time every day to center myself."

- *Measurable:* For example, instead of saying we will get centered generally, we can describe how we will measure the experience of centering. This may be by measuring changes in mood or stress. We could also measure the number of minutes per day we are centering ourselves.

- *Achievable, Realistic, and Time-bound:* For example, instead of saying, "I will not be stressed again because I will know how to be centered," we can shift into a more achievable goal: "I want to reduce my stress level by 10 percent in the next five weeks."

As you can see, outcomes serve as the mile-markers on the journey of going from our current state of priorities (location) to arriving at our desired destination (of our future state). Much like you would break a trip up into different sections, the outcomes can be phased over time as short, mid-, and long term. The outputs, then, are the mile-markers, ways to measure where we actually are relative to where we want to go. Much like a GPS tells us where we are when we are lost on a trip, outputs help us to check in with how far we have come from the location, and how close we are to arriving at our desired destination (vision of our future state).

Step 5: Intervention activities—"Choose the best route for the journey"

The next step in the planning process is to determine which road you will take to get from here (priorities) to there (future state). This is the section of planning that most people think is the entire program plan—the place where we decide what we will include in the program. However, this step is best completed only after we have a strong understanding of our current state (priorities) and future state (vision). When these are well defined, we can get a better understanding of the multiple routes we can take to get from here (priorities) to there (vision). We can then choose the route that is best aligned; it ideally addresses or solves problems in our current state, and also takes us towards our desired outcomes and vision in the future state.

Although there are many ways to think about (conceptualize), design, and develop a yoga program, I prefer to consider the "5 Ws" when designing a yoga program. These are the central components needed in a program design.

Who:

- Who is the program for? What do we know about the client's priorities and goals?
- Who will support the client in engaging with the program? (Peers? Providers?)
- Who is the best yoga professional to deliver the program?

Why:

- Why does the client want to commit to the program? (Their vision of impact?)
- Why can't the client miss out on the program? (Opportunity cost)

When:

- When will the program begin and end? (How long do we have for the program?)

- When can the client complete the program during their day? (Daytime? Evening?)

- When will the client check in on their progress to goals?

Where:

- Where can the client practice? (Location—online? In person?)

- Where can the client bring yoga into their day off the mat? (Work? Home?)

What:

- What will the program include—off the mat? (Dinacharya, to follow the knowledge of the day, or daily health routine? Social support?)

- What will the program include—on the mat? (Sadhana, personal practice? Other practices?)

- What will the program exclude? (What does the client need to stop doing to support program goals? What does the client need to let go of to commit?)

How we can co-create a Yoga for One program: the Frequency, Intensity, Time, Type-Volume, Progression (FITT-VP) framework

The FITT-VP framework from the field of exercise science is used to create effective and individualized fitness plans. While it is often applied in the design and co-creation of cardiovascular and strength training programs, it can also be adapted for co-creating a yoga practice program to ensure it meets the specific needs and goals of an individual. Here's how you can use FITT-VP in the context of a yoga practice program:

Frequency (number of practices per week):

- Determine how often the individual will practice yoga. This could be daily, a few times a week, or on specific days.

- Consider the individual's current fitness level, time availability, and overall goals when deciding on frequency.

Intensity (cardiovascular challenge level):

- In yoga, intensity can be related to the level of effort put into practice. For example, a strenuous vinyasa practice focused on postures will have a higher intensity than a meditation class or restorative session.

- It is important to tailor the intensity based on the individual's fitness level and goals, and to adjust this based on their other physical activity throughout the week. For example, an avid runner is already meeting their weekly requirement for cardiovascular activity when they are running, therefore, they do not need to consider the cardiovascular (intensity) level of their yoga practices to optimize their health. They may want to choose more gentle practices (from a cardiovascular intensity perspective), such as yin and restorative. On the other hand, a client with diabetes who is not otherwise physically active will need a practice that has more intensity to align with medical guidance that suggests that they need 150 minutes of cardiovascular activity per week at a low–moderate level.

Time (duration):

- Determine the length of each yoga session. Sessions can range from 15 minutes to an hour or more, depending on the individual's schedule and goals.

- Consider factors like attention span, physical endurance, and the time available for practice when setting the duration.

Type (mode of yoga):

- Choose the style or type of yoga that aligns with the individual's goals and preferences. Options include hatha, vinyasa, Ashtanga, yin, or restorative yoga, among others. As noted under "Intensity," the type of yoga selected should also consider the individual's physical condition and any specific needs or restrictions they may have.

Volume (total amount):

- Determine the total workload or volume of the yoga program. This involves the combination of frequency, duration, and the number of poses or sequences.

- Calculate the weekly or monthly volume to ensure that it aligns with the individual's goals and provides a balanced practice.

Progression (advancement):

- Plan for gradual progression in the yoga program to prevent plateaus and encourage ongoing improvement.

- Progression might involve adding new poses, increasing the intensity or duration of sessions, or refining alignment and technique over time.

Incorporating the FITT-VP principle into a yoga practice program allows for customization and adaptation to an individual's specific needs and goals. It ensures that the yoga program is neither too easy nor too challenging, promoting a safe and effective practice. Regular monitoring and adjustments based on progress are also essential to keep the program aligned with the individual's evolving needs and objectives. Please remember, however, that FITT-VP is generally applied to physical activity program design; yoga practice program design includes much more than physical postures.

Step 6: Inputs—"Pack for the trip"

In the final step of the program planning and evaluation process we consider what we need for a successful trip. These are inputs—a combination of the client's resources such as their resilience and readiness. We want to be sure that we are ready to take the trip, that we are resilient enough to handle its anticipated challenges and packed with the right resources so as not to have the journey end too soon. I encourage folks using this logic model to note that if we don't feel that we have what we need for success of the intervention (one-on-one yoga program), we need to either solve that problem (i.e., acquire the needed inputs) or rethink the program's structure. If you don't have the inputs you need for successful activities (program), then you are encouraged to rework the logic model until you know you have the right inputs in place for a successful journey.

Please remember as you use this logic model template that it is not meant to be a script. Much like we might adapt a yoga pose for the unique mind–body–heart–system of a human, we can do the same with this logic model template. Allow it to inspire your work with those receiving care—but don't let this tool get in the way of what will organically happen when you connect with your client and engage in the co-creation process.

CONCLUSION

One of the helpful benefits of using this Yoga for One logic model as a shared decision-making and co-creation tool is that it keeps us in a facilitative role rather than a prescriptive one. The act of prescribing a program to a person is much different than partnering with them to facilitate (and co-create) it. Here the yoga professional is co-creating with the client—they are partners with equal power. That said, the logic model's real-life applications will emerge differently depending on the yoga professional's scope of practice.

Here are a few examples of how various yoga professional roles impact our work with the Yoga for One logic model for program co-creation:

- *Allied health referral:* If the client's problems and/or priorities are beyond the scope of yoga facilitation (in any role), and/or if a screening is needed to determine the severity of the problem/s, the yoga facilitator refers the client to the appropriate allied health provider/s.

- *Yoga therapist:* If the client needs a customized plan of care to be developed in order to address their priorities and realize their vision, then the person is best served by yoga therapy. In this scenario, the yoga therapist partners with the individual to co-create a Yoga for One practice program, on or off the mat. This process includes the design, delivery, and evaluation of the program plan, which includes yoga philosophy, postures, and practices.

- *Yoga mentor:* If the client would benefit from being mentored in the process of deepening their understanding of the philosophy, postures, and/or practices of yoga, or they need support in implementing their yoga therapy plan of care, then yoga mentoring is suggested. Generally a mentor works with other professionals, although this is not always the case.

- *Yoga teacher:* If the client would benefit from learning more about yoga philosophy, yoga practices, and/or yoga postures to begin their journey or to address their priorities, realize their vision, or deepen their understanding of yoga, they would benefit from yoga education in a class, a small group, or one-on-one setting. This is the type of setting that is most commonly found in studios and other community health settings—and is most often how people in the Western world are introduced to yoga. In the ideal scenario, a yoga student attends classes that are part of an overall strategic program or plan of care—so that they are relevant and have lower risk.

- *Yoga coach:* If the client would benefit from support in behavior change for lifestyle modification and/or facilitated awareness of their personal barriers to taking care of themselves on or off the mat, yoga coaching is recommended. Here the yoga coach engages in both talk- and movement-based coaching, encouraging the client to explore their mindsets and their somatic awareness. Yoga coaching can be integrated into yoga classes, yoga mentoring, or yoga therapy, or it can be offered as a separate option.

As you can see, logic models offer us a simple tool for co-creating a yoga practice program with our clients. The six steps of logic modeling enable us to get strategic about how the program can take the client from where they are today (priorities for health, wellness, and well-being) to where they want to go (future state), by planning out the journey from today to tomorrow. We also learned how we can develop a practice program that is aligned with SMART goals, and that is grounded in the reality of our current inputs (resources). In the next chapter, we will explore how you can create a practice that fits within this bigger program picture while staying present with your clients. Let's go there next!

CHAPTER 7

Aligning Daily Practices to the Program Needs and Goals

INCLUSIVE STRATEGIES

In the first chapter of this book, I shared several assumptions that we would be making on this journey. One of these is that you are a yoga professional. And because I am assuming that you are a yoga professional, this means that you are already familiar with practice design. I am therefore focusing this chapter on illustrating how you can match practice components (such as philosophy, postures, pranayama, or other practices) to the client's needs based on the data you collected in the intake, interview, and assessment process. The idea here is that I want you to remember that the practice design is best grounded in the data you receive from the client (as discussed in Chapter 5), and refined based on the parameters of their program logic model (as explored in Chapter 6).

MEDICAL CONCERNS

In this section, we explore general considerations for modifying practices based on common medical concerns. These are general in nature and should not be misconstrued as medical advice. Please be sure that you are following the client's allied health professional guidance, and encouraging them to listen to their own inner guidance (intuition and interoception) as well. It is important for one-on-one yoga professionals to stay within their scope of practice—do not work with a client with significant medical challenges unless you have formal training in doing so. Remember to ask your client to seek medical approval before working with you, and to remind them to keep you informed of any changes to their medical status or healthcare treatment plan (from allied health providers).

Nervous system concerns

- *Function:* Responsible for transmitting signals between different parts of the body. It includes the central nervous system (brain and spinal cord) and the peripheral nervous system.

- *Common medical concerns:* Multiple sclerosis, Parkinson's disease, Alzheimer's disease, epilepsy, neuropathies.

- *Practice accommodations:*

  - *Intensity—low to moderate:* Emphasize gentle and restorative yoga practices that don't overstimulate the nervous system. Avoid intense, physically demanding poses or practices that may lead to increased cognitive load and/or mental stress.
  - *Time—session duration:* 20–60 minutes. Adapt the duration based on individual needs and energy levels.
  - *Types of yoga practice:* Restorative and yin yoga—focus on deep relaxation and gentle stretching to calm the nervous system. Hatha yoga—incorporate slow-paced, mindful asana practice with an emphasis on alignment. Yoga nidra—deep relaxation and guided meditation to reduce stress and anxiety. Pranayama—breathing techniques to regulate the nervous system. Mindfulness meditation to enhance mental clarity and reduce stress. Mudra—hakini mudra to support brain function and concentration.

Cardiovascular system concerns

- *Function:* Responsible for pumping and circulating blood throughout the body. It includes the heart and blood vessels.

- *Common medical concerns:* Heart disease, hypertension (high blood pressure), arrhythmias, coronary artery disease.

- *Practice accommodations:*

  - *Intensity—low to moderate:* Emphasize gentle and controlled movements in yoga poses to avoid excessive strain on the heart. Incorporate restorative and relaxation practices to manage stress, which can contribute to cardiovascular issues. Avoid vigorous or strenuous practices that may elevate heart rate and blood pressure to unsafe levels.
  - *Time—session duration:* 20–60 minutes. Offer options for shorter or longer

sessions based on individual fitness levels and preferences. Warm-up and cool-down periods should be included in each session.

- *Types of yoga practice:* Hatha yoga—focus on gentle, slow-paced asana practice with an emphasis on alignment and breath awareness. Restorative yoga—incorporate supported poses and deep relaxation to reduce stress and promote cardiovascular recovery. Gentle yoga—include poses suitable for individuals with limited mobility or specific cardiovascular concerns. Pranayama—teach controlled breathwork techniques to improve respiratory function and reduce stress. Meditation—use mindfulness meditation to promote relaxation and mental clarity. Mudra—ganesha mudra to remove emotional stress and tension.

Respiratory system concerns

- *Function:* Responsible for taking in oxygen and expelling carbon dioxide. It includes the lungs, bronchi, trachea, and other respiratory passages.

- *Common medical concerns:* Asthma, chronic obstructive pulmonary disease (COPD), pneumonia, bronchitis.

- *Practice accommodations:*

  - *Intensity—low to moderate:* Emphasize slow and controlled movements to avoid overexertion. Encourage participants to listen to their bodies and avoid pushing themselves too hard. Incorporate restorative practices to reduce stress, which can exacerbate respiratory symptoms.
  - *Time—session duration:* 20–60 minutes. Offer flexibility in session length to accommodate varying energy levels and physical conditions. Include gentle warm-up and cool-down periods to prepare and relax the respiratory muscles.
  - *Types of yoga practice:* Pranayama—focus on breath control exercises to strengthen the respiratory muscles and improve oxygenation. Hatha yoga—emphasize slow and controlled movements with attention to alignment and breath awareness. Gentle yoga—include poses suitable for individuals with limited mobility and respiratory challenges. Restorative yoga—utilize supported postures and deep relaxation to enhance respiratory ease. Mudra—prana mudra to encourage balance in the vayus.

Musculoskeletal system concerns

- *Function:* Provides structure and support to the body, allowing for movement. It includes bones, muscles, tendons, ligaments, and joints.

- *Common medical concerns:* Osteoarthritis, rheumatoid arthritis, osteoporosis, muscle strains, and fractures.

- *Practice accommodations:*

  - *Intensity—low to moderate:* Prioritize gentle and mindful movements to avoid strain or exacerbating existing conditions. Emphasize the importance of listening to the body and practicing within individual pain thresholds.
  - *Time—session duration:* 20–60 minutes. Adapt session length to the individual's physical condition and comfort level. Incorporate a well-balanced combination of poses and relaxation techniques to maximize benefits.
  - *Types of yoga practice:* Hatha yoga—focus on slow, controlled movements, proper alignment, and breath awareness. Gentle yoga—incorporate poses suitable for individuals with limited mobility and musculoskeletal issues. Yin yoga—utilize passive stretches held for longer durations to target deep connective tissues. Restorative yoga—emphasize relaxation and rejuvenation through supported poses. Mudra—prithvi mudra sukhasana to connect to the earth element and foster balance with groundedness.

Digestive system concerns

- *Function:* Responsible for breaking down food into nutrients and waste. It includes the stomach, intestines, liver, and pancreas.

- *Common medical concerns:* Gastroesophageal reflux disease (GERD), irritable bowel syndrome (IBS), Crohn's disease, ulcerative colitis.

- *Practice accommodations:*

  - *Intensity—low to moderate:* Prioritize gentle yoga practices to avoid excessive strain or discomfort. Emphasize relaxation and mindful movements to reduce stress, a common trigger for digestive issues.
  - *Time—session duration:* 20–45 minutes. A shorter practice focused on targeted poses and techniques can be more accessible and sustainable for individuals with digestive concerns. Ensure that there is adequate time for relaxation and stress reduction within the session.
  - *Types of yoga practice:* Hatha yoga—incorporate gentle, well-aligned poses

that promote relaxation and stimulate digestion. Restorative yoga—utilize supported poses and props to encourage deep relaxation and relieve tension. Pranayama—integrate breathwork techniques that calm the nervous system and aid digestion, such as diaphragmatic breathing and alternate nostril breathing. Mudra—apana mudra to balance digestion.

Endocrine and lymphatic system concerns

- *Functions:*

  - Endocrine: produces hormones that regulate metabolism, growth, and development
  - Lymphatic: maintains fluid balance, produces white blood cells, and filters harmful substances.

- *Common medical concerns:* Diabetes, hypothyroidism, lymphedema.

- *Practice accommodations:*

  - *Intensity—low to moderate:* Prioritize gentle and restorative yoga practices to avoid overexertion. Focus on relaxation, stress reduction, and gentle movements to support hormonal balance and lymphatic flow. As the client becomes stronger, and with medical approval, encourage increases in strength and flexibility to support the client in finding hormonal balance.
  - *Time—session duration:* 30–60 minutes. A longer practice allows for a comprehensive approach to supporting endocrine and lymphatic health. Ensure that there is adequate time for relaxation and breathwork within the session.
  - *Types of yoga practice:* Hatha yoga—incorporate gentle, well-aligned poses to stimulate endocrine glands and encourage lymphatic circulation. Restorative yoga—utilize supported poses and props to promote deep relaxation and reduce stress, which can affect endocrine function. Yin yoga—focus on long-held, passive stretches to target deep tissues and stimulate lymphatic flow. Pranayama—include breathwork techniques that support relaxation and hormonal balance, such as abdominal breathing and Bhramari (Bee Breath). Mudra—garuda mudra (eagle gesture) to balance and activate energy flow throughout the body.

Reproductive system concerns

- *Function:* Responsible for producing offspring and regulating sex hormones in both males and females.

- *Common medical concerns:* Polycystic ovary syndrome (PCOS), endometriosis, prostate issues.

- *Practice accommodations:*

  - *Intensity—low to moderate:* Prioritize gentle and restorative yoga practices to avoid overexertion. Focus on relaxation, stress reduction, and gentle movements to support hormonal balance and lymphatic flow.
  - *Time—session duration:* 35–60 minutes. A longer practice allows for a comprehensive approach to supporting endocrine and lymphatic health. Ensure that there is adequate time for relaxation and breathwork within the session.
  - *Types of yoga practice:* Hatha yoga—incorporate gentle, well-aligned poses to stimulate endocrine glands and encourage lymphatic circulation. Restorative yoga—utilize supported poses and props to promote deep relaxation and reduce stress, which can affect endocrine function. Yin yoga—focus on long-held, passive stretches to target deep tissues and stimulate lymphatic flow. Pranayama—include breathwork techniques that support relaxation and hormonal balance, such as abdominal breathing and Bhramari (Bee Breath). Mudra—yoni mudra to promote harmony in the organs.

Integumentary system concerns

- *Function:* Acts as a barrier to protect the body from the outside environment. It includes the skin, hair, nails, and sweat and oil glands.

- *Common medical concerns:* Eczema, acne, psoriasis, skin cancer.

- *Practice accommodations:*

  - *Intensity—low to moderate:* Gentle to moderate-intensity yoga practices are suitable for promoting skin health without overexertion. Focus on relaxation and stress reduction to prevent skin-related issues caused or exacerbated by stress.
  - *Time—session duration:* 35–60 minutes. A longer practice allows for a comprehensive approach to skin health and overall well-being. Include relaxation and mindfulness practices within the session for stress reduction.

    – *Types of yoga practice*: Hatha yoga—incorporate poses that improve blood circulation and gently stimulate the skin's surface. Vinyasa yoga—utilize flowing sequences to enhance overall circulation and vitality. Restorative yoga—focus on relaxation and stress reduction. Mudra—varun mudra for connection with water (hydration). Pranayama—practice breath techniques that are calming and cooling so as to promote healthy function of the integumentary system.

WELL-BEING ACCOMMODATIONS

In this section we will explore how you can enhance the well-being experience for each practice within your client's Yoga for One program. For example, if your client has set a goal for their Yoga for One program to improve their physical well-being, because their WHO-5 score is low on the "feeling active and vigorous" dimension, you could design each practice within the program to focus on physical well-being enhancement. This approach is similar to the way you would tune into a radio station. We wouldn't try to listen to all stations at once; instead we would tune into one station at a time. In a similar way, we can encourage the client to "tune in" to the well-being dimension that they are focusing on for their program, through the experience of each practice within the program. Let's explore strategies you can take to support each practice from a well-being outcome perspective. You'll notice that in each section, we are encouraging the client to engage in the co-creation process, by asking them to share with you what would work best for them.

Physical well-being

Clients who wish to focus on physical well-being for their Yoga for One program may be doing so because they had a low score on the WHO-5 "I have felt active and vigorous" question, and/or because they wish to improve their overall physical health and wellness profile. As we meet them where they are in this intention, we can focus our efforts on practice choreography and cueing to enhance their experience of their physical well-being. Essentially, we would focus the practice on the needs of their physical (gross) body, in keeping with annamaya kosha.

Practice Strategies: After welcoming the client to the session, ask them to share where in their body they would like to focus the day's practice—in terms of their low body, mid body, or upper body. Ask them if they have any physical goals for the session, such as "to feel stronger in my upper body" or to "feel more open in my hips". This is a different way to get at whether they feel their body is not quite right today (i.e. tight, stiff, weak)—by framing it based on their desired outcome for the session.

Begin with a gentle warm-up sequence, including Marjaryasana-Bitilasana (Cat–Cow Pose), Balasana (Child's Pose), and Adho Mukha Svanasana (Downward Facing Dog), focusing on the client's experience of their annamaya kosha. Ask them to share how they feel in their body as they move through space, and create the shapes of the asanas. You can also ask them to share their physical experience of other yoga practices, such as pranayama (breathing techniques) and/or mudras. Here they are tuning into their physical well-being, and we are encouraging them to make the adjustments they need to feel good in their body. Then, we can modify future practices, or possibly the program, accordingly.

Social well-being

Clients who wish to focus on their social well-being (and their sense of connection) for their Yoga for One program, may be doing so because they had a low score on the WHO-5 "I woke up feeling refreshed and rested" question, and/or because they wish to improve their overall social health and wellness profile. As we meet them where they are in this intention, we can focus our efforts on practice choreography and cueing to enhance their experience of their social well-being, and their overall sense of vitality (energy). Essentially, we would focus the practice on responding to the needs of their energy level, in keeping with pranamaya kosha.

Practice Strategies: After welcoming the client to the session, ask them to share where they feel in terms of their overall energy level. Ask them to rate if they want to leave the session more energized, less energized, or about the same. This is a different way to get at whether they feel their energy is too high or too low—by framing it based on their desired outcome for the session.

Based on their response, share practices and postures according to their energy goals. If they want to feel more energized by the end of the practice, encourage heart-opening poses like Bhujangasana (Cobra Pose) and Urdhva Mukha Svanasana (Upward Facing Dog). If they want to feel less energized (more calm and grounded) then offer them postures that bring their heart to the earth (such as child's pose or forward fold). If they want to feel about the same in terms of energy level, offer them a practice that is generally balanced from an open front body vs open back body perspective, with some twists to help them to stay connected to their internal energy.

Mental well-being

Clients who wish to focus on their mental well-being (and their mental experience of peace, focus, and clarity) for their Yoga for One program, may be doing so because they had a low score on the WHO-5 "I have felt calm and relaxed" question, and/or because they wish to improve their overall mental health and wellness profile. As we meet them where they are in this intention, we can focus our efforts on practice choreography and cueing to enhance their experience of their mental well-being, and their overall sense of emotional regulation, which I personally define as their ability to maintain a sense of equanimity even as life hands them good and bad plot twists (such as the stress of struggle and the stress of success). Essentially, we would focus the practice on responding to the needs of their mental well-being, in keeping with manomaya kosha.

Practice Strategies: After welcoming the client to the session, ask them to share where they feel in terms of their overall mental state. Ask them to share if they would like you to focus the session on their achievement of mental clarity and/or mental calm. This is a different way to get at whether they feel their mental state is too agitated or too foggy—by framing it based on their desired outcome for the session.

Based on their response, share practices and postures according to their mental clarity and/or calming state goals. If they want to feel more clear by the end of the practice, encourage a combination of inverted postures such as adho mukha svanasana (downward facing dog) and centering practices such as mudras. If they want to feel more calm mentally by the end of the practice, combine postures that bring their heart to the earth (such as child's pose or forward fold) with pranayama (breath) practices that focus on apana vayu (release work) and samana vayu (centering work). After you have led them through the practices, ask them to share, if they are comfortable, whether they have achieved their desired state of calm and/or clarity. Then, ask them if they have any ideas for what would help them to continue working towards achieving these goals, and/or continue the experience of these states in the rest of their day. In the case of mental well-being, it is important to engage in this choice talk, as part of shared decision-making after the practice and not before, in order to not overwhelm them mentally.

Purpose well-being

Clients who wish to focus on their purpose well-being (and their mental experience of peace, focus, and clarity) for their Yoga for One program, may be doing so because they had a low score on the WHO-5 "My daily life has been filled with things that interest me" question, and/or because they wish to improve their overall sense of meaning and purpose. As we meet them where they are in this intention, we can focus our efforts on practice choreography and cueing to enhance their connection to their internal sense of purpose and their dharma. Essentially, we would focus the practice on responding to the needs of their purpose well-being, which connects their own individual and unique sense of dharma with their dedication to serving the world, in keeping with the aims of vijnanamaya kosha.

Practice Strategies: After welcoming the client to the session, ask them to share where they feel in terms of their overall sense of meaning and purpose. Ask them to share if they would like you to focus the session on providing space for them to connect to their inner sense of purpose and meaning. This approach will especially help those who do not feel they have found their sense of meaning and purpose yet because the focus is not on their achievement of finding their purpose but instead on exploring what it might be.

Based on their response, share practices and postures giving them space to explore their inner world, and their sense of deeper Truth. For example, you might begin with a gentle warmup of postures to help them to shift their attention from the outside world into their interior experience. Then, as they become more mindful of how they are moving "from the inside out," we can shift to providing them stillness for the body and time for contemplation. Restorative postures work especially well here, because they are not asking for any "work" from the body and they are providing physical support (through props) and the experience of being held. Here, the client can ideally access a feeling of physical and mental safety. While they are in an open-hearted restorative posture, you can ask them to expand their thinking of the possibilities for their purpose.

After you have led them through the practices, ask them to share what they discovered about their purpose when they had the space and time to go deep within their awareness. Then, ask them if they have any ideas for what would help them to continue working towards exploring their purpose further (if they are trying to find it) or applying their purpose (if they already know what it is).

Emotional well-being

Clients who wish to focus on their emotional well-being (and their experience of joy, bliss, and spirit) for their Yoga for One program, may be doing so because they had a low score on the WHO-5 "I have felt cheerful and in good spirits" question, and/or because they wish to improve their overall experience of joy in life. As we meet them where they are in this intention, we can focus our efforts on practice choreography and cueing to enhance their connection to their internal sense of consciousness, and the ways that their light (of joy) connects to their sense of spirit (whether it is a zest for living and/or a connection to a higher power or divinity) and their connection to the greater good (their connection to the world around us). Essentially, we would focus the practice on responding to the needs of their emotional well-being, which connects their own individual and unique sense of joy to the overall expansion of the consciousness and spirit of the world, in keeping with the aims of anandamaya kosha.

Practice Strategies: After welcoming the client to the session, ask them to share where they feel in terms of their overall sense of joy and spiritual connection. Ask them to share if they would like you to focus the session on supporting them into connection with the light they have within them. This approach will especially help those who feel burned out in their light, overwhelmed by what the world is asking them, so much so that they have forgotten that the light of consciousness shines within them.

Based on their response, share practices and postures giving them space to explore their inner sense of joy and fun, as well as their sense of creativity. For example, you might begin with a gentle warmup of postures to help them to shift their attention from the outside world into their interior experience. Then, as they become more comfortable, you might ask them how they can make a posture silly or more fun today. As they find ways to express joy through the silliness of a posture, they are breaking through the mental and cultural barriers that are putting a "lamp shade" on their light. They are given encouragement to connect to what is true for them, and to feel free to express themselves, even if it is through a simple yoga posture variation. In this way we are encouraging the client to access their sense of self-liberation and joy—to access their true yoga within.

After you have led them through the practices, ask them to share what they discovered in this practice, and where they want to take it next (into their day, week, or year). As they share with you what this means for the future, encourage them to remember that their light is uniquely theirs, and that they have it within them no matter what is happening in the outside world. And, encourage them to remember that their light of joy will "shine" that much more brightly for others (becoming contagious to them), as they continue to take care of their other layers (koshas) of well-being.

GUNAS

The gunas represent the fundamental qualities that shape our physical, mental, and emotional states. Recognizing and balancing these energies through tailored yoga practices is a crucial element in the design of one-on-one yoga programs. We can co-create yoga practices that specifically target the equilibrium of sattva, rajas, and tamas in individuals. By tailoring the choice of asanas (physical postures), pranayama (breathing techniques), and meditation practices to balance these energies, yoga instructors and practitioners can harmonize the mind, body, and spirit, ultimately leading to a more holistic and personalized yoga experience.

- Balancing sattva:

  - *Asanas:* Gentle flows like Surya Namaskar (Sun Salutations) or calming poses such as Sukhasana (Easy Pose), Padmasana (Lotus Pose), and Savasana (Restorative Pose).
  - *Pranayama:* Techniques like Anulom Vilom (Alternate Nostril Breathing) and Brahmari (Bee Breath) to maintain balance and harmony.
  - *Meditation:* Guided meditations or self-inquiry techniques to deepen their sense of self-awareness.

- Balancing rajas:

  - *Asanas:* Start with dynamic asanas to channel their active energy, such as vinyasa flow or Ashtanga sequences, and then transition to grounding poses like Balasana (Child's Pose) or Pachimottanasana (Seated Forward Bend).
  - *Pranayama:* Techniques like Sheetali (Cooling Breath) or deep, controlled Ujjayi (Victorious Breath) can help calm an overactive mind.
  - *Meditation:* Guided relaxation or mindfulness practices to help them focus and calm their mind.

- Balancing tamas:

  - *Asanas:* Energizing sequences such as Surya Namaskar (Sun Salutations) or poses that improve circulation and energy like Navasana (Boat Pose), or the Virabhadrasana series (Warrior Poses).
  - *Pranayama:* Bhastrika (Bellows Breath) or Kapalbhati (Skull Shining Breath) to increase energy and dispel lethargy.
  - *Meditation:* Dynamic meditations or ones focusing on cultivating inner fire and motivation.

DOSHAS

Yoga, with its holistic approach to well-being, harmoniously complements Ayurveda, the ancient Indian system of medicine. In Ayurveda, doshas represent an individual's unique blend of physical and mental characteristics. Tailoring an individual's yoga practice according to their dosha can optimize benefits, creating balance and harmony within. Let's explore the recommended yoga practices for each dosha type.

- Vata practices:

  - *Calming and grounding asanas:* Vrikshasana (Tree Pose), Virabhadrasana II (Warrior II), Balasana (Child's Pose)
  - *Meditation and pranayama:* Guided meditation, Nadi Shodhana (Alternate Nostril Breathing).

- Pitta practices:

  - *Cooling and relaxing asanas:* Chandra Namaskar (Moon Salutation), Ustrasana (Camel Pose), Paschimottanasana (Seated Forward Bend)
  - *Meditation and pranayama:* Meditative practices focused on compassion, Shitali Pranayama (Cooling Breath).

- Kapha practices:

  - *Stimulating and energizing asanas:* Surya Namaskar (Sun Salutations), vinyasa flows, Navasana (Boat Pose), Dandasana (Plank Pose)
  - *Pranayama:* Bhastrika (Bellows Breath) (invigorating).

- Vata–pitta or pitta–vata practices:

  - *Combination of calming and cooling poses:* Half Ardha Matsyendrasana (Lord of the Fishes Pose), Salamba Sarvangasana (Supported Shoulder Stand)
  - *Breathing and meditation:* Deep breathing exercises with periods of meditative reflection.

- Pitta–kapha or kapha–pitta practices:

  - *Combination of relaxing and energizing sequences:* Bhujangasana (Cobra Pose), Matsyasana (Fish Pose)
  - *Pranayama:* Alternating between calming and stimulating pranayama techniques.

- Kapha–vata or vata–kapha practices:

  - *Grounding and invigorating sequences:* Utkatasana (Chair Pose), Supta Matsyendrasana (Supine Twist)
  - *Pranayama:* Incorporating both energizing and calming pranayama practices.

SOCIAL DETERMINANTS OF HEALTH

Yoga can play a supportive role in addressing the social determinants of health by promoting mental and emotional well-being, reducing stress, and fostering a sense of community and connection. Here are some yoga practice recommendations that can be beneficial:

- *Community yoga classes:* Encourage individuals to participate in community-based yoga classes. These not only provide the physical benefits of yoga, but also offer a sense of belonging and social interaction.

- *Mindfulness and stress reduction:* Incorporate mindfulness meditation and stress reduction techniques into yoga practice. These can help individuals manage stress related to the social determinants of health, such as financial difficulties or housing instability.

- *Group yoga sessions:* Organize group yoga sessions in community centers or local parks to promote social interaction and a sense of community among participants.

- *Partner yoga:* Partner yoga poses and exercises can enhance social connections. Practicing yoga with a partner or in pairs can foster trust, communication, and cooperation.

- *Yoga for mental health:* Offer yoga classes specifically designed to address mental health challenges associated with the social determinants of health. These can focus on emotional regulation, anxiety reduction, and improving mood.

- *Yoga for trauma:* Provide trauma-informed yoga classes that create a safe and supportive environment for individuals who have experienced trauma related to the social determinants of health.

- *Yoga for self-care:* Teach yoga practices that promote self-care and self-compassion, which are essential for individuals facing stressors related to social determinants.

- *Breathwork (pranayama):* Incorporate pranayama techniques like deep breathing exercises, which can help individuals manage stress, anxiety, and emotional well-being.

- *Yoga philosophy:* Share yoga philosophy and principles related to compassion, non-judgment, and community support. Discuss how these principles can be applied in daily life to improve social connections and well-being.

- *Gratitude practice:* Include a gratitude or loving-kindness meditation at the end of yoga sessions to encourage clients to focus on positive aspects of their lives and foster a sense of gratitude for their community and support systems.

- *Volunteer opportunities:* Promote volunteerism and community engagement as part of a holistic approach to addressing social determinants. Encourage clients to get involved in community service projects.

- *Group discussions:* After yoga sessions, provide opportunities for group discussions on topics related to the social determinants of health. This can create a supportive space for individuals to share their experiences and challenges.

- *Access to yoga resources:* Ensure that individuals have access to affordable or free yoga resources, including classes, online videos, and written materials, to support their well-being.

As we can see, yoga can be adapted based on the social determinants of health, as a valuable tool for promoting mental and emotional resilience, fostering social connections, and improving overall well-being in individuals facing challenging circumstances.

LIFESTYLE MEDICINE

Lifestyle medicine focuses on the impact of lifestyle choices on health and well-being. Yoga, with its holistic approach, can be an integral part of a lifestyle medicine plan. Here are some yoga practice recommendations that align with lifestyle medicine principles:

- *Nutrition awareness:* Encourage mindful eating practices and body awareness through yoga. Incorporate yoga poses that emphasize core engagement, balance, and awareness of the breath. Encourage clients to consider what other "food" they are taking into their bodies through their choices (environmental factors).

- *Physical activity:* Promote physical activity and fitness through yoga asanas. Develop yoga sequences that target strength, flexibility, and cardiovascular health. Surya Namaskar (Sun Salutations) and vinyasa flows are excellent for building endurance and improving overall fitness.

- *Stress reduction:* Integrate stress reduction techniques into yoga practice. Practices like deep breathing exercises (pranayama) and restorative yoga poses like Savasana (Restorative Pose) and Balasana (Child's Pose) can help reduce stress and promote relaxation.

- *Sleep hygiene:* Teach yoga practices that support healthy sleep patterns. Gentle bedtime yoga sequences, relaxation techniques, and yoga nidra can aid in improving sleep quality.

- *Social connection:* Organize group yoga classes or community yoga events to promote social connections and a sense of belonging. Encourage clients to interact and support each other. Discuss healthy communication and relationship building within the context of yoga philosophy. Encourage clients to apply principles like compassion, non-judgment, and empathy in their relationships.

- *Tobacco and alcohol awareness:* Use yoga as a platform to raise awareness about the harmful effects of tobacco and excessive alcohol consumption. Explore yoga's role in supporting individuals in making healthier choices.

Lifestyle medicine and yoga share a common goal of promoting well-being through healthy lifestyle choices. By integrating yoga practices that align with lifestyle medicine principles, individuals can cultivate a balanced and sustainable approach to health and wellness.

KOSHAS

As we have learned, the kosha framework helps us to understand the relationship between the body, energy, mind, heart, and spirit: "The imagery often used to demonstrate the concept of kosha is the layers of an onion that may be peeled away from each other. The pancamaya model implies something quite different, however: that these five dimensions are all present, all the time, in each part of the human system, even in each cell of the body. They cannot be 'peeled' apart; they are inseparable from each other."[25]

We will now explore specific practices that aim to address imbalances in each kosha. Please keep in mind that although we are discussing healing practices for one kosha at a time, these practices will have a ripple effect on the other koshas as well. Let's explore the following:

- Annamaya kosha: Saririka Chikitsa = healing using the body

- Pranamaya kosha: Prana Chikitsa = healing using prana

- Manomaya kosha: Indriya Chikitsa = healing through the senses

- Vijnanamaya kosha: Manasika Chikitsa = healing using the mind

- Anandamaya kosha: Adhyatmika Chikitsa = healing from the core.

Annamaya kosha: Saririka Chikitsa

The annamaya kosha layer is the sheath related to the physical body, and Saririka Chikitsa is healing using the body. According to Desikachar, Bragdon, and Bossart (2005),[26] the practice of five types of asanas can support healing.

Samasthiti (Equal Standing)

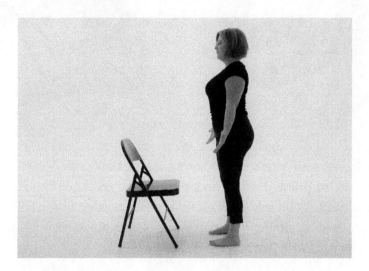

The spine in these postures is erect, or vertical, in a neutral, healthy alignment. The benefits of Samasthiti include:

- *Improved posture:* Practicing Samasthiti helps in aligning the body correctly from head to toe. It encourages a straight and neutral spine, which can lead to improved posture over time.

- *Body awareness:* This pose fosters a heightened sense of body awareness. As you stand still and focus on alignment, you become more attuned to how your body feels and its subtle movements.

- *Grounding:* The pose encourages a sense of grounding and connection with the earth. This grounding effect can help reduce feelings of anxiety and restlessness.

- *Preparation for other poses:* Samasthiti serves as a starting point for many yoga sequences and asanas (poses). It prepares the body and mind for transitions into other standing poses, forward bends, and Surya Namaskar (Sun Salutations).

Pascimatana

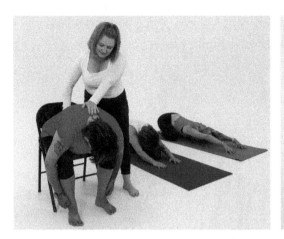 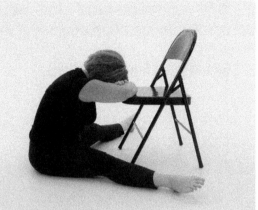

The Sanskrit term *pascimatana* means "stretching the back of the body," and involves yoga postures that primarily focus on stretching the posterior or back side of the body. These can help improve flexibility, alleviate tension in the back and hamstrings, promote relaxation, and support emotional release. Here are some common postures associated with Pascimatana:

- *Paschimottanasana (Seated Forward Bend):* This involves extending your legs in front of you and folding forward at the hips to reach for your toes or shins. It stretches the entire posterior chain, including the spine, hamstrings, and calves.

- *Uttanasana (Standing Forward Bend):* In Uttanasana, you stand with your feet hip-width apart and hinge forward at the hips, reaching for your toes or the floor. This pose stretches the hamstrings and lower back while also promoting relaxation.

- *Janu Sirsasana (Head-to-Knee Forward Bend):* In this seated pose, one leg is extended while the sole of the opposite foot is placed against the inner thigh. You then fold forward over the extended leg, reaching for the toes. It provides a deep stretch to the hamstrings and lower back.

- *Upavistha Konasana (Wide-Angle Seated Forward Bend):* In this seated pose, you spread your legs wide apart and fold forward from the hips, reaching for the floor or your feet. It stretches the inner thighs, hamstrings, and lower back.

- *Supta Padangusthasana (Reclining Hand-to-Big-Toe Pose):* This is a reclined posture where you lie on your back, raise one leg, and hold on to the big toe with your hand. It provides a gentle stretch to the hamstrings and lower back.

- *Balasana (Child's Pose):* While not a forward bend in the traditional sense, this involves kneeling with your knees apart and sitting back on your heels, reaching your arms forward and resting your forehead on the mat. It's a restful posture that gently stretches the lower back and promotes relaxation.

- *Adho Mukha Svanasana (Downward Facing Dog):* This is a full back-body stretch, especially for the low back, gluteals, and hamstrings.

Purvatana

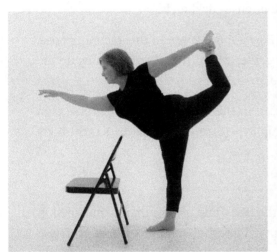 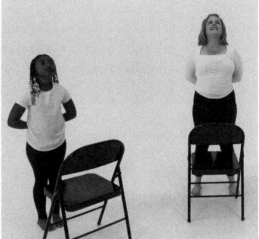

The Purvatana postures focus on stretching the front of the body. They help open up the chest and engage the back body muscles. Here are some common yoga poses that fall under the category of Purvatana:

- *Urdhva Mukha Svanasana (Upward Facing Dog):* This involves lifting the chest and upper body off the ground while keeping the legs and pelvis on the mat. It stretches the front of the body, strengthens the arms and back, and supports posture.

- *Bhujangasana (Cobra Pose):* This is a gentle backbend that stretches the front of the torso and strengthens the back muscles. It can help alleviate stiffness in the low back.

- *Ustrasana (Camel Pose):* This is a deep backbend that stretches the entire front of the body, from the chest to the thighs. It is excellent for opening the heart center and promoting emotional release.

- *Dhanurasana (Bow Pose):* In this pose, you grasp your ankles and lift your chest and thighs off the ground, resembling the shape of a bow. It stretches the entire front body, including the abdomen and hip flexors.

- *Virabhadrasana I (Warrior I Pose):* While primarily a standing pose, this involves lifting the arms overhead, which stretches the front of the torso and promotes expansion.

- *Anjaneyasana (Low Lunge):* This pose involves a deep lunge with one foot forward and the other extended behind. It stretches the front hip flexors and can be a preparatory pose for more intense backbends.

- *Supta Baddha Konasana (Reclining Bound Angle Pose):* In this reclining pose, the soles of the feet are brought together while lying down, opening up the hips and stretching the front of the torso.

- *Nataraasana (Lord of the Dance Pose):* In this standing pose, the torso is in a backbend and the back leg is in hip hyperextension, creating a front-body stretch.

Parivritti

The Parivritti postures involve twisting the body, and are commonly included in yoga practices to improve spinal flexibility, digestion, and detoxification. These poses typically engage the core and help release tension in the back, making them beneficial for overall spinal health. Here are some common Parivritti postures:

- *Parivritta Trikonasana (Revolved Triangle Pose):* In this pose, you stand with your feet apart, and as you twist, one hand reaches for the opposite foot while the other extends upward. It is an intense stretch for the hamstrings, and a deep twist for the spine.

- *Parivritta Parsvakonasana (Revolved Side Angle Pose):* Similar to Parivritta Trikonasana, this involves bending the front knee while twisting and reaching one arm to the floor and the other towards the ceiling.

- *Parivritta Ardha Chandrasana (Revolved Half Moon Pose):* This pose combines balancing on one leg with a twist. You reach one hand to the floor while the other extends upward, and your body forms a "T" shape.

- *Parivritta Janu Sirsasana (Revolved Head-to-Knee Pose):* In this seated twist, you bend one leg and place the foot against the inner thigh of the extended leg. You then twist your upper body towards the bent knee.

- *Bharadvajasana (Bharadvaja's Twist)*: This seated twist involves sitting with your legs extended, bending one knee, and twisting your upper body towards the bent knee. It's excellent for releasing tension in the lower back.

- *Marichyasana C (Marichi's Pose C)*: A seated twist that combines leg binding with a deep spinal twist. One leg is extended, and the other is bent, with the foot placed close to the hip.

- *Parivritta Utkatasana (Revolved Chair Pose)*: This standing twist is a variation of Utkatasana, where you twist your upper body to one side while maintaining the chair-like squat position.

- *Parivritta Baddha Parsvottanasana (Revolved Bound Side Angle Pose)*: This pose combines a forward bend with a twist. One leg is forward in a lunge position, and you twist your torso to one side while binding your hands behind your back.

- *Parivritta Supta Padangusthasana (Revolved Reclining Hand-to-Big-Toe Pose)*: In this supine pose, you lie on your back and bring one knee towards your chest. You then extend the bent leg to the side while twisting your torso in the opposite direction.

- *Parivritta Hasta Padangushthasana (Revolved Standing Hand-to-Big-Toe Pose)*: In this standing pose, you begin in Hasta Padangushthasana (Big Toe Forward) and then revolve to hold the foot with the opposite hand. Flexibility in the hamstrings and low back is required for neutral spine.

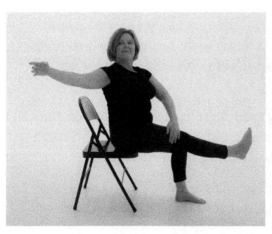 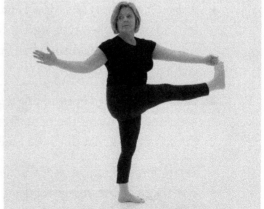

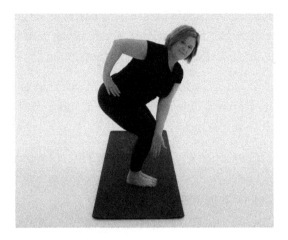

Parsva

These postures involve taking the torso to one side. These also engage the core and can help release tension in the side body. Here are some common Parsva postures:

- *Parsvakonasana (Extended Side Angle Pose):* In this pose, you step your feet wide apart and bend one knee, creating a lunge. The hand of the bent knee side rests on the floor or a yoga block, while the other arm reaches overhead, creating a lateral stretch.

- *Parsvottanasana (Pyramid Pose):* This pose involves standing with one foot forward and the other foot turned inward. You fold forward at the hips, bringing your chest towards your front knee, creating a lengthening sensation along the back of the extended leg.

- *Ardha Chandrasana (Half Moon Pose):* In this balancing pose, you stand on one leg and extend the other leg out to the side while simultaneously reaching the same-side hand towards the floor and lifting the other hand towards the ceiling.

- *Parsva Balasana (Thread the Needle Pose):* Start in a tabletop position, then slide one arm under the opposite arm, creating a twisting motion through the spine. Note that this pose is also a twisting pose (Parivritti).

- *Parsva Virabhadrasana (Side Warrior Pose):* Similar to Virabhadrasana II (Warrior II), this pose involves a deep lunge, but you extend one arm overhead, creating a lateral stretch.

- *Parsva Bakasana (Side Crow Pose):* This is an advanced arm balance where you twist your torso to one side while balancing on your hands.

- *Parsva Upavistha Konasana (Side Seated Wide-Angle Forward Bend)*: In this seated pose, you have your legs wide apart, and you bend to one side, reaching for your toes on that side.

- *Parsva Dhanurasana (Side Bow Pose)*: This pose is a variation of Dhanurasana in which you bend one knee and reach for the foot on that side, creating a side stretch.

- *Parsva Sukhasana (Sideways Easy Pose)*: In this seated pose, cross your legs, and then twist the upper body to one side, creating a gentle spinal twist.

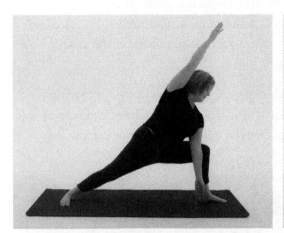 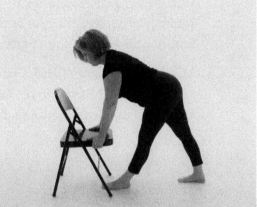

Pranamaya kosha: Prana Chikitsa

Prana Chikitsa, often translated as healing using prana, is a fundamental aspect of yoga that involves harnessing and manipulating the vital life force energy known as "prana" for the purpose of healing and holistic well-being. Prana is believed to be the subtle energy that animates all living beings and connects the physical body to the mind and spirit. In yoga philosophy, prana flows through the body along energy pathways called "nadis," and is concentrated in energy centers known as "chakras."

Prana Chikitsa encompasses a wide range of practices aimed at balancing and optimizing the flow of prana throughout the body. These practices include:

- *Pranayama:* The conscious control and regulation of the breath. Through various breathing techniques, individuals can influence the movement of prana in the body. Pranayama practices can calm the mind, energize the body, and enhance the overall flow of prana.

- *Mudras:* Hand gestures or positions that can influence the flow of prana in the body. By holding specific hand positions, individuals can direct prana to different areas of the body and stimulate specific energy pathways.

- *Bandhas:* Energetic locks or seals created within the body by contracting specific muscles. These locks can control the flow of prana and prevent it from escaping the body. Common bandhas include mula bandha (root lock), uddiyana bandha (abdominal lock), and jalandhara bandha (throat lock).

- *Visualization:* Visualization techniques involve mentally directing prana to specific areas of the body for healing or revitalization. This practice combines focused intention with the subtle flow of energy to promote healing and balance.

- *Chakra activation:* Energy centers located along the spine, each associated with specific qualities and functions. Practitioners can use meditation, visualization, and energy awareness techniques to activate and balance the chakras, ensuring the smooth flow of prana.

- *Mantras and chanting:* Certain sounds and syllables, when chanted or repeated as mantras, are believed to resonate with pranic energy. Chanting mantras can help clear energy blockages, balance the mind, and enhance pranic flow.

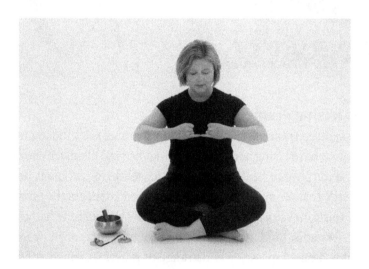

The vayus are vital components of Prana Chikitsa (healing using prana) in yoga, and play a significant role in understanding and working with the subtle flow of prana (life force energy) within the body. In yogic philosophy, vayus are considered the "winds" or subtle forces responsible for the movement and distribution of prana. There are five primary vayus, each with its distinct functions and locations in the body:

- *Apana aayu:* The area below the navel, associated with the lower abdomen and pelvic region. Its primary functions include the elimination of waste, reproductive processes, and fertility. In terms of healing, apana vayu relates to the process of purification and removal of toxins from the body. Practices focused on exhalation and the engagement of uddiyana bandha (abdominal lock) and mula bandha (root lock) can help balance and heal apana vayu.

- *Samana vayu:* The area of the belly around the navel. It governs the process of digestion and assimilation of nutrients. Samana vayu is essential for ensuring proper digestion and absorption of food, which is crucial for overall health. Healing practices related to samana vayu involve equal ratio breath control and the engagement of uddiyana bandha (abdominal lock).

- *Prana vayu:* The chest and heart region. It is responsible for mental functions, thoughts, and emotions. In the context of healing, prana vayu relates to enhancing mental well-being and clarity. Pranayama techniques focusing on inhalation, such as deep, controlled breathing, help activate and balance prana vayu.

- *Udana Vayu:* The throat region. It influences communication, expression, and the movement of prana upward. In terms of healing, udana vayu is associated with the use of sound and vibration. Chanting, singing, and vocal practices are utilized to balance and heal udana vayu. The practice of jalandhara bandha (throat lock) can also be beneficial.

- *Vyana vayu:* This is unique among the vayus as it is present throughout the entire human system, facilitating the circulation of prana throughout the body. Healing practices related to vyana vayu often involve the use of mudras, which are hand gestures that direct prana to specific areas. Mudras can help balance and harmonize the overall flow of prana within the body.

Prana Chikitsa also relates to a holistic approach to healing that recognizes the importance of the chakras in maintaining overall health and balance. By working with the chakras through specific practices and techniques, individuals can enhance the flow of prana, address health issues, and promote well-being on multiple levels—physical, mental, emotional, and spiritual. Here's how Prana Chikitsa and chakras are interconnected:

- *Balancing prana through chakras:* In Prana Chikitsa, one of the fundamental principles is the understanding that prana flows through the nadis and is regulated by the chakras. Each chakra is associated with certain types of pranic energy and specific aspects of physical and mental health. When prana is balanced and flows freely through these energy centers, it supports overall well-being.

- *Activation and healing:* Prana Chikitsa involves techniques to activate, cleanse, and balance the chakras. Various practices such as specific pranayama exercises, visualizations, meditation, and asanas (yoga poses) can be used to direct prana to specific chakras, remove blockages, and restore their optimal functioning. The goal is to ensure that each chakra is open and spinning at the right speed, which contributes to a harmonious flow of energy throughout the body.

- *Correspondence with health:* Each chakra is associated with certain physical organs, psychological attributes, and emotional states. When imbalances occur in a particular chakra, it can manifest as physical or emotional health issues. Prana Chikitsa practitioners work to identify and address these imbalances through techniques that focus on the specific chakra or chakras involved.

- *Overall healing:* The balanced flow of prana through the chakras not only supports physical health but also contributes to mental and emotional well-being. As prana moves through the chakras, it can help release emotional blockages, reduce stress, and promote mental clarity and emotional stability.

When chakras are disturbed, it can manifest as imbalances in the body, mind, and emotions. To bring them back into balance, specific yoga practices can be employed. Here are some yoga program recommendations for each of the chakras when they are disturbed.

- Root chakra (muladhara)—grounding and stability:

  - Asanas: Tadasana (Mountain Pose), Virabhadrasana I (Warrior I), and Vrksasana (Tree Pose)
  - Pranayama: deep, grounding breaths, emphasizing the exhale
  - Meditation: visualize a vibrant red, glowing light at the base of the spine
  - Bija: chant or silently repeat the mantra "Lam."

- Sacral chakra (svadhisthana)—emotions and sensuality:

  - Asanas: Baddha Konasana (Bound Angle Pose), Parivrtta Trikonasana (Revolved Triangle Pose), and Dhanurasana (Bow Pose)
  - Pranayama: slow and deep breathing, emphasizing the exhale
  - Meditation: visualize a bright orange light at the sacrum

- Bija: chanting or silent repetition of the mantra "Vam."

- Solar plexus chakra (manipura)—personal power and confidence:

    - Asanas: Navasana (Boat Pose), Ustrasana (Camel Pose), and Bhujangasana (Cobra Pose)
    - Pranayama: Kapalabhati (Breath of Fire) and diaphragmatic breathing
    - Meditation: visualize a radiant yellow light at the solar plexus
    - Bija: chant or silently repeat the mantra "Ram."

- Heart chakra (anahata)—love and compassion:

    - Asanas: Urdhva Dhanurasana (Upward Bow Pose), Matsyasana (Fish Pose), and Ardha Uttanasana (Half Forward Bend)
    - Pranayama: heart-centered breathing and Anulom Vilom (Alternate Nostril Breathing)
    - Meditation: visualize a warm, green light at the heart center
    - Bija: chanting or silent repetition of the mantra "Yam."

- Throat chakra (vishuddha)—communication and expression:

    - Asanas: Setu Bandha Sarvangasana (Bridge Pose), Halasana (Plow Pose), and Matsyendrasana (Seated Twist)
    - Pranayama: Ujjayi (Victorious Breath) and chanting of "Om"
    - Meditation: visualize a soothing blue light at the throat
    - Bija: chant or silently repeat the mantra "Ham."

- Third eye chakra (ajna)—intuition and insight:

    - Asanas: Balasana (Child's Pose), Janu Sirsasana (Head-to-Knee Forward Bend), and Garudasana (Eagle Pose)
    - Pranayama: Nadi Shodhana (Alternate Nostril Breathing) and deep, mindful breathing
    - Meditation: visualize an indigo light at the space between the eyebrows
    - Bija: chanting or silent repetition of the mantra "Om" or "Aum."

- Crown chakra (sahasrara)—spiritual connection and unity:

    - Asanas: Padmasana (Lotus Pose), Sirsasana (Headstand), and Savasana (Restorative Pose)
    - Pranayama: breath awareness and Sahaja Pranayama (natural breath)
    - Meditation: visualize a radiant violet or white light at the crown of the head
    - Bija: chant or silently repeat the mantra "Aum" or "Ah."

Manomaya kosha: Indriya Chikitsa

Indriya Chikitsa, the healing of the senses, involves practices aimed at refining and nurturing our sensory experiences. These are designed to enhance awareness, self-control, and conscious perception. Here are some key practices of Indriya Chikitsa:

- *Yama and niyama:* The ethical and moral principles of yoga, known as yama and niyama, form the foundation of Indriya Chikitsa. These principles include ahimsa (non-harming), satya (truthfulness), asteya (non-stealing), brahmacharya (moderation), aparigraha (non-attachment), saucha (cleanliness), santosha (contentment), tapas (discipline), svadhyaya (self-study), and ishvara pranidhana (surrender to a higher force). Practicing yama and niyama helps cultivate self-awareness and self-control.

- *Trataka:* This practice involves focused gazing, typically on a specific point or object. It sharpens the sense of sight and concentration. It can include gazing at a candle flame, a point on the wall, or an image. Trataka enhances visual perception and develops inner focus.

- *Nada yoga:* This is the yoga of sound and involves practices aimed at refining the sense of hearing. These include listening to soothing music, mantras, or the internal sound within the body, such as the heartbeat or the sound of the breath. Nada yoga enhances auditory perception and fosters inner harmony.

- *Eka rasa ahara:* This practice involves consuming only one particular taste for a specified period, such as eating only sweet or sour foods for a set duration. Eka rasa ahara helps refine the sense of taste and brings awareness to our dietary choices.

- *Mauna vrata:* Mauna vrata is a vow of silence, practiced to develop control over the sense of speech. During this practice, individuals refrain from speaking and communicate through non-verbal means. Mauna vrata enhances awareness of verbal communication patterns and fosters inner stillness.

- *Pratyahara:* Pratyahara, often referred to as withdrawal of the senses, is the practice of consciously redirecting the senses inward. It involves cutting off external sensory inputs and focusing the mind on inner experiences. Practices like trataka, nada yoga, and meditation contribute to the development of pratyahara.

- *Meditation:* Various meditation techniques are integral to Indriya Chikitsa.

Meditation cultivates mindfulness, self-awareness, and conscious perception. Techniques like mindfulness meditation, vipassana, and trataka meditation are commonly employed to refine the senses.

- *Svadhyaya:* One of the niyamas, svadhyaya involves self-study and self-reflection. Journaling, contemplation, and introspection are practices that fall under svadhyaya. This self-inquiry fosters awareness of an individual's thoughts, emotions, and behaviors.

These practices of Indriya Chikitsa collectively contribute to heightened sensory perception, self-awareness, and the ability to consciously direct and control an individual's sensory experiences. By refining the senses, individuals can navigate the external world with greater clarity and inner balance.

Vijnanamaya kosha: Manasika Chikitsa

Manasika Chikitsa, which focuses on healing using the mind, involves practices aimed at cultivating mental clarity, emotional balance, and spiritual insight. These practices harness the power of the mind to promote holistic well-being. Here are some key practices of Manasika Chikitsa:

- *Bhavana (visualization):* Bhavana refers to the practice of visualization, where individuals mentally create and dwell on specific images, objects, or experiences. This technique can be used for various purposes, such as visualizing healing energy, positive outcomes, or inner qualities like love and compassion.

- *Affirmations:* These are positive statements that individuals repeat to themselves to reinforce desired beliefs or qualities. By regularly practicing affirmations, an individual can shift their thought patterns and cultivate a positive mindset. For example, repeating affirmations about self-worth or inner peace can be part of Manasika Chikitsa.

- *Metta (loving-kindness) meditation:* Metta meditation is a practice of generating feelings of love and goodwill towards oneself and others. It involves silently repeating phrases like "May I [or others] be happy, may I be healthy," and so on. This practice promotes emotional well-being, compassion, and mental clarity.

- *Mindfulness meditation:* This involves paying non-judgmental attention to the present moment, including thoughts, emotions, bodily sensations, and the surrounding environment. It enhances self-awareness, emotional regulation, and mental focus.

- *Cognitive restructuring:* This practice involves identifying and challenging negative thought patterns and replacing them with more positive and realistic ones. It is often used to address conditions like anxiety and depression, and helps individuals develop a healthier perspective on their experiences.

- *Japa (mantra repetition):* Japa is the repetition of a mantra or sacred word. Mantras are repeated either aloud or silently to calm the mind, deepen concentration, and connect with higher states of consciousness. Common mantras include "Om," "So Hum," or personalized affirmations.

- *Mindful eating:* This involves being fully present and aware while consuming food. It encourages individuals to savor each bite, pay attention to flavors and textures, and eat with gratitude. This practice can promote a healthier relationship with food and reduce overeating.

- *Journaling:* Keeping a journal is a valuable tool for self-reflection and self-expression. Through journaling, individuals can explore their thoughts, emotions, and experiences, gaining insights into their inner world and fostering mental clarity.

- *Guided imagery:* This involves listening to recorded scripts or visualizations that guide individuals through relaxing and healing mental journeys. It can be used to reduce stress, manage pain, and promote emotional healing.

- *Chakra meditation:* This focuses on the energy centers within the body known as chakras. By meditating on each chakra, individuals can balance their energy and promote mental and emotional well-being.

- *Yama and niyama:* The ethical and moral principles of yoga, yama and niyama guide an individual's behavior and mindset. Practicing satya (honesty), santosha (contentment), and tapas (self-discipline) are examples of how these principles contribute to mental healing.

These practices of Manasika Chikitsa empower individuals to cultivate a positive and resilient mindset, nurture emotional well-being, and deepen their understanding of the mind's potential for healing and transformation. By incorporating these practices into their daily lives, individuals can achieve greater mental clarity, emotional balance, and spiritual growth.

Anandamaya kosha: Adhyatmika Chikitsa

Adhyatmika Chikitsa, which focuses on healing from the core or the spiritual dimension, involves practices aimed at deepening an individual's spiritual connection, self-realization, and inner transformation. These practices go beyond the physical and mental realms and delve into the core of an individual's being. Here are some key practices of Adhyatmika Chikitsa:

- *Ishvara pranidhana (surrender to a higher force):* This practice involves surrendering ego and personal will to a higher power or divine force. It fosters humility, acceptance, and a sense of trust in a greater cosmic order. Ishvara pranidhana helps individuals let go of the need to control everything and find inner peace.

- *Shraddha (faith):* Cultivating faith in a higher force, whether it's a deity, the universe, or a spiritual principle, is a fundamental aspect of Adhyatmika Chikitsa. Shraddha provides solace and resilience in times of suffering and uncertainty.

- *Yajna (ritual):* Yajna refers to a set of actions or techniques performed with mindfulness and a specific intention. Rituals can vary widely but often involve offerings, chanting, and symbolic gestures. They are performed to connect with the divine, purify the Self, and create a sacred space.

- *Satsang (spiritual community):* Satsang involves gathering with like-minded individuals who are on a spiritual path. It provides a supportive and nurturing environment for spiritual growth, self-reflection, and the exchange of wisdom.

- *Seva (selfless service):* Engaging in acts of selfless service, without expecting anything in return, is a way to transcend ego and for the individual to connect with the core of their being. Seva helps individuals develop compassion, humility, and a sense of interconnectedness with all living beings.

- *Mauna vrata (silence and solitude):* Mauna vrata is a vow of silence that allows individuals to turn their attention inward. It helps quiet the chatter of the mind, enhances self-awareness, and deepens the connection to the inner self.

- *Svadhyaya (sacred text study):* Svadhyaya is the practice of studying sacred texts and scriptures. It involves self-examination, introspection, and contemplation of spiritual teachings for an individual to gain insight into their true nature and the nature of reality.

- *Meditation on symbols and archetypes:* This practice involves meditating on specific symbols, deities, or archetypes that hold spiritual significance. It can facilitate a deeper understanding of universal truths and archetypal energies within the psyche.

- *Prayer and mantras:* Engaging in prayer or chanting of mantras (sacred sounds or words) can be a powerful way to connect with the divine and invoke spiritual blessings. Mantras are often used to focus the mind and elevate consciousness.

- *Pilgrimage and sacred journeys:* Visiting sacred places, temples, or natural sites of spiritual significance is a way to immerse oneself in a sacred and transformative environment. Pilgrimage can deepen spiritual connection and provide a sense of renewal.

- *Contemplative practices:* Contemplative practices involve deep reflection on spiritual themes or questions. Through contemplation, individuals can gain insights into their own spiritual journey and the nature of existence.

Adhyatmika Chikitsa invites individuals to explore the depths of their spiritual nature, seek higher truths, and experience a profound connection with the divine. These practices encourage inner transformation, self-realization, and the realization of the interconnectedness of all life.

CONCLUSION

In this chapter, and throughout this book, we have explored how yoga philosophy, practices, and postures can be tailored for one-on-one yoga clients, in inclusive and evidence-informed ways. I congratulate you on finishing the journey that is this book, and thank you for your commitment to your clients. The world needs people who care enough to support other people with their own self-care and self-liberation. Because ultimately, we are all one. Namaste!

About the Author

Suzie Carmack, PhD, MFA, MEd, ERYT 500, NBC-HWC, PCC, C-IAYT, is a board-certified health coach, certified yoga therapist, and well-being scholar. As the Department Chair of Yoga Therapy and Ayurveda at the Maryland University of Integrative Health, she directs and teaches in the world's only accredited Master of Science degree program in Yoga Therapy. She is also a Senior Scholar for the Center for the Advancement of Well-Being at George Mason University, where she develops evidence-informed training programs and interventions to advance healthcare and public health workforce well-being. Dr. Carmack is the author of two #1 best-sellers dedicated to raising the yoga literacy of the public: *Well-Being Ultimatum* (2015) and *Genius Breaks* (2017), and is a chapter author in *Embracing Complexity in Health* (Springer, 2019) and *Weight Loss for Life* (Hopkins University Press, 2022). She has also authored numerous peer-reviewed journal articles and is regularly commissioned to co-create and evaluate evidence-informed programs for government agencies and organizations in the public and private sectors. As the CEO and founder of YogaMedCo, LLC, she has trained 1000s of yoga coaches, yoga teachers, yoga personal trainers, and organizational leaders in her evidence-informed methodology, bringing the practices of yoga, lifestyle medicine, and coaching together. Learn more about Dr. Carmack and how you can join her efforts to move the world to well-being at www.DrSuzieCarmack.com

Endnotes

1   Sullivan, M. B. and Hyland Robertson, L. C. (2020) *Understanding Yoga Therapy: Applied Philosophy and Science for Health and Well-Being.* Abingdon: Routledge.

2   Desikachar, K., Bragdon, L., and Bossart, C. (2005) "The yoga of healing: Exploring yoga's holistic model for health and well-being." *International Journal of Yoga Therapy 15,* 1, 17–39, p.20.

3   See www.drsuziecarmack.com

4   Owen, K. L., Watkins, R. C., and Hughes, J. C. (2022) "From evidence-informed to evidence-based: An evidence building framework for education." *Review of Education 10,* 1, e3342.

5   Sullivan, M., Finlayson, D., and Moonaz, S. (2017) "Understanding yoga's roots in evidence-informed practice." *Yoga Therapy Today,* 40–42.

6   Chaturvedi, S., Kumar, N., Tillu, G., and Patwardhan, B. (2021) "Research, biomedicine and Ayurveda: From evidence-based medicine to evidence-informed healthcare." *Indian Journal of Medical Ethics VI,* 4, 301–305.

7   AIFS (Australian Institute of Family Studies) (no date) "What is an evidence-informed approach to practice and why is it important?" https://aifs.gov.au/resources/short-articles/what-evidence-informed-approach-practice-and-why-it-important

8   IATY (International Association of Yoga Therapists) (2019) "Contemporary definitions of yoga therapy."

9   CDC (Centers for Disease Control and Prevention) (2022) "The socio-ecological model: A framework for prevention." Violence Prevention. www.cdc.gov/violenceprevention/about/social-ecologicalmodel.html

10 Litchfield, L., Perryman, K., Avery, A., Campbell, S., Gill, P., and Greenfield, S. (2021) "From policy to patient: Using a socio-ecological framework to explore the factors influencing safe practice in UK primary care." *Social Science & Medicine 277,* 113906.

11 Elwyn, G., Tilburt, J., and Montori, V. (2013) "The ethical imperative for shared decision-making." *European Journal for Person Centered Healthcare 1,* 1, 129–131.

12 Feuerstein, G. (2012) *The Yoga Tradition: Its History, Literature, Philosophy and Practice.* Chino Valley, AZ: Hohm Press, pp.342–352.

13 Jorgenson, E. (2015) "Why value creation is the foundation of business: How to define it, measure it, and manage it." Blog, September 14. www.ejorgenson.com/blog/value-creation

14 NSMC (National Social Marketing Centre) (no date) "What is social marketing?" www.thensmc.com/content/what-social-marketing-1

15 McDonough-Means, S. I., Kreitzer, M. J., and Bell, I. R. (2004) "Fostering a healing presence and investigating its mediators." *Journal of Alternative & Complementary Medicine 10,* Supplement 1, S-25, abstract.

16 Drossman, D. A., Chang, L., Deutsch, J. K., Ford, A. C., *et al.* (2021) "A review of the evidence

and recommendations on communication skills and the patient–provider relationship: A
Rome foundation working team report." *Gastroenterology 161*, 5, 1670–1688.

17 All names used in this book are pseudonyms, to protect anonymity.

18 Topp, C. W., Østergaard, S. D., Søndergaard, S., and Bech, P. (2015) "The WHO-5 Well-Being Index: A systematic review of the literature." *Psychotherapy and Psychosomatics 84*, 3, 167–176.

19 Dervin, B. and Foreman-Wernet, L. (2012) "Sense-Making Methodology as an Approach to Understanding and Designing for Campaign Audiences." In R. E. Rice and C. K. Atkin (eds) *Public Communication Campaigns* (4th edn) (pp.147–161). Abingdon: SAGE Publications Ltd.

20 Carmack, S. (2014) "Making Sense of Well-Being: A Mixed-Methods Study Applying Sense-Making Theory to Explore the Role of Communication Competence and Social Support in Physical, Emotional, Mental and Comprehensive Well-being." Doctoral dissertation, George Mason University.

21 Dervin, B. (2011) as cited in Reinhard, C. D. and Dervin, B. (2012) "Comparing situated sense-making processes in virtual worlds: Application of Dervin's Sense-Making Methodology to media reception situations." *Convergence 18*, 1, 27–48.

22 Carmack, S. and Mikeska, D. (2021) *Yoga Personal Trainer Training* by YogaMedCo [Training Manual].

23 Travis, J.W. (2007) "Key concept #1: The illness–wellness continuum." The Wellspring. www.thewellspring.com/wellspring/introduction-to-wellness/357/key-concept-1-the-illnesswellness-continuum.cfm.html

24 Pearson, N., Naylor, P. J., Ashe, M. C., Fernandez, M., Yoong, S. L., and Wolfenden, L. (2020) "Guidance for conducting feasibility and pilot studies for implementation trials." *Pilot and Feasibility Studies 6*, 1–12.

25 Desikachar, K., Bragdon, L., and Bossart, C. (2005) "The yoga of healing: Exploring yoga's holistic model for health and well-being." *International Journal of Yoga Therapy 15*, 1, 17–39, p.17.

26 Desikachar, K., Bragdon, L., and Bossart, C. (2005) "The yoga of healing: Exploring yoga's holistic model for health and well-being." *International Journal of Yoga Therapy 15*, 1, 17–39.